Cookin

D0735457

Prostate
Health

641.5631 Cou

Courtier, M.
Prostate health.

PRICE: $9.00 (anf/m)

Marie-Annick Courtier

Foreword by Lauren Feder, M.D.

Cooking Well: Prostate Health

Text copyright © 2011 Marie-Annick Courtier

Hatherleigh Press is committed to preserving and protecting the natural resources of the Earth. Environmentally responsible and sustainable practices are embraced within the company's mission statement.

Hatherleigh Press is a member of the Publishers Earth Alliance, committed to preserving and protecting the natural resources of the planet while developing a sustainable business model for the book publishing industry.

This book was edited and designed in the village of Hobart, New York. Hobart is a community that has embraced books and publishing as a component of its livelihood. There are several unique bookstores in the village. For more information, please visit www.hobartbookvillage.com.

DISCLAIMER
This book offers general cooking and eating suggestions for educational purposes only. In no case should it be a substitute nor replace a healthcare professional. Consult your healthcare professional to determine which foods are safe for you and to establish the right diet for your personal nutritional needs.

Courtier, Marie-Annick.
  Cooking well. Prostate health / Marie-Annick Courtier.
      p. cm. -- (Cooking well)
  ISBN 978-1-57826-376-9 (pbk.)
  1. Prostate--Diseases--Diet therapy. 2. Prostate--Diseases--Prevention. 3. Men--Nutrition. 4. Cookbooks. I. Title. II. Title: Prostate health.
  RC899.C68 2011
  641.5'631--dc22
                        2010051951

www.hatherleighpress.com

Cover Design by Nick Macagnone
Cover Photography by Catarina Astrom
Interior Design by Nick Macagnone

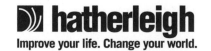

hatherleigh
Improve your life. Change your world.

Table of Contents

Foreword   v

Chapter 1: The Importance of Maintaining a Healthy Prostate   1

Chapter 2: How the Right Diet Can Help   5

Chapter 3: Dietary Suggestions for a Healthy Lifestyle   11

Chapter 4: The Recipes   17
    Breakfast   19
    Soups & Salads   35
    Fish & Seafood Entrées   59
    Meat, Poultry & Vegetable Entrées   77
    Side Dishes & Snacks   95
    Desserts   115

References   132

Acknowledgments

Hatherleigh Press would like to extend a special thank you to June Eding—without your hard work and dedication this book would not have been possible.

Foreword

According to the Mayo Clinic, half of all men in their sixties exhibit signs and symptoms of prostate enlargement. As our lifespan increases, conditions of the prostate will affect nearly all men sooner or later. With a plethora of information available on the Internet and in books, patients are savvier than ever before. In addition to standard medical treatments for benign prostatic hypertrophy (BPH) and prostate cancer, many people are interested in how exercise, spirituality, lifestyle, and nutrition can benefit men suffering with these conditions.

According to Dr. Henry Bieler, "Food is your best medicine." Many men and their families are interested in taking a proactive approach to prostate health, and this wonderful book *Cooking Well: Prostate Health* provides a sound foundation. Readers will appreciate the concise and thorough overview of the prostate, and the chapter on dietary suggestions for a healthy lifestyle offers superb tips on what to eat and how to eat. Despite the fact that this book is geared towards prostate health, both men and women will benefit greatly from the recipes. The ingredients in the recipes are fresh and pleasing to the palate, and will appeal to men and their families as this little gem remains true to its title in providing over 100 easy and delicious recipes for prostate management. Eating well begins with cooking well.

In good health,
—*Lauren Feder, M.D.*

Chapter 1

The Importance of Maintaining a Healthy Prostate

The prostate (from the Greek prostates, "one who stands before", "protector", or "guardian") is a gland of the male reproductive system. The prostate stores and produces *prostatic fluid*. This fluid is released along with other male reproductive fluids and helps to ensure successful reproduction. Prostate function is regulated by male hormones, including testosterone. The prostate surrounds the urethra and is located just below the bladder. In a healthy human man, the prostate is slightly larger than a walnut.

As a man ages and the production of testosterone and other hormones increases, the prostate naturally gets larger. However, in some individuals the body can create an excess of prostate cells and the prostate will get too large. An enlarged prostate can block the urethra, leading to bladder and kidney infections, as well as other health problems. Inflammation of the prostate gland is a condition known as *prostatitis*.

Prostatitis

There are four main types of *prostatitis*. Two uncommon forms, *acute prostatitis* and *chronic bacterial prostatitis,* can be treated with antibiotics. Another less common form of prostatitis, known as *category IV prostatitis*, is a type of leukocytosis (a condition where there is a raised white blood cell count in the bloodstream). The most common kind of prostatitis is *benign prostatic hyperplasia (BPH).* BPH rarely causes symptoms before the age of 40, but as a man gets older BPH becomes increasingly common; more than half of men in their sixties show signs of BPH, whereas as many as 90% of men in their seventies and eighties have symptoms. BPH can progress from early symptoms to a more serious condition.

Symptoms of BPH include frequent urination and weak urinary stream. If left untreated, bladder stones can form and bacteria can build up in the bladder, causing a urinary tract infection. Some patients who have chronic urinary retention as a result of BPH can even develop renal failure (kidney failure).

As stated, the odds of contracting BPH rise drastically as a man ages. Generally, the risk of BPH increases roughly 4 percent each year after the age of 55. By age 60, the odds increase to 50 percent and, by 85, the odds jump up to 95 percent.

The chance of developing prostatitis is one reason why, as the years go by, it is increasingly important for men to continue to lead a healthy lifestyle in order to guard prostate health.

Prostate Cancer

Prostate cancer is one of the most common forms of cancer for older men. Prostate cancer occurs when cells in the prostate gland multiply at an abnormally high rate. There are often no symptoms of prostate cancer in the early stages. Treatments include surgery, chemotherapy, cryotherapy, hormonal therapy and/or radiation. Anyone diagnosed with prostate cancer should work closely with their doctor to determine what kind of treatment is necessary or if a "watchful waiting" approach, to take time to observe if the cancer progresses, is advisable.

Although the exact causes of prostate cancer are unknown, studies show that middle aged and older American males are most likely to be diagnosed with a malignant form of prostate cancer. Worldwide, close to half a million new cases of prostate cancer are diagnosed each year. Almost half of these cases will occur in the United States. Furthermore, one out of six American men is at risk of developing prostate cancer. This risk increases for men over the age of 50. This makes prostate cancer, next to lung and skin cancer, the most common cancer to afflict the American male population.

Leading a Healthy Life

In addition to increased risk as a man ages, obesity is a major contributor to whether or not someone develops BPH or prostate cancer. Generally, if a man gains more than 3 pounds each year between the ages of 25 and 50, the odds of developing prostate cancer increase by 50%. This means that men of all ages must develop good diet and exercise habits in order to prevent long-term weight gain and maintain a healthy prostate.

There are certain factors that can help prevent an enlarged prostate. These factors are related to both diet and lifestyle choices. Those who have a lower risk of BPH and prostate cancer are characterized by a lack of belly fat, a commitment to exercise/physical activity, regular consumption of five or more servings of fruits and vegetables each day, and a low-fat diet.

Good habits should be maintained throughout a man's life in order to prevent any future prostate-related problems. Eating healthful foods and maintaining a regular exercise regimen is vital. To reduce the risk of BPH or prostate cancer, take the following steps:

- Exercise
- Avoid obesity by keeping fat intake low
- Eat fruits and vegetables and make responsible food choices
- Choose specific nutrient-rich foods (see the next chapter)

A key component to maintaining a healthy lifestyle is eating well. In the next chapter we will take a closer look at how making the right food choices can help to encourage a healthy prostate.

Chapter 2

How the Right Diet Can Help

Eating well and taking good care of yourself makes a big difference in helping to prevent an enlarged prostate and guard prostate health. Incorporating more nutrient-rich fresh fruits and vegetables into your diet is key, and certain foods are especially beneficial (more details can be found later in this chapter). However, just as important as making the right eating choices is making the effort to avoid the wrong ones.

Making the Right Choices

No matter what your age or family history, developing good habits when it comes to eating and exercise can never start too soon. Use the guidelines in this book to help you stick with a regular meal and exercise plan. If you slip up, make every effort to get back on track. Guarding your health and preventing painful and costly prostate-related problems later in life is worth the effort it takes now.

Remember to speak to your doctor about the dietary guidelines below and seek his or her guidance based on your own unique symptoms and needs before beginning any diet regimen.

Basic Nutrition

Take steps to drastically reduce or eliminate specific foods, listed below, from your diet.

- **REMOVE** artificial ingredients, additives, and chemicals from your regular diet. This includes cutting out processed foods, preservatives, chemicals, and artificial sweeteners.

- **AVOID** fried, fatty, highly caloric, and processed foods.

- **ALSO AVOID** refined sugar, excessive caffeine and alcohol consumption, junk/fast food, unnecessary drugs, non-organic foods, and any other foods high in sugar, fat, and cholesterol.

Keep in mind that eliminating any products that you are accustomed to using will take time. If you would like to cut something out of your diet for good, be sure to avoid it for at least a month. This will reduce your cravings and make the habit easier to maintain over the long term.

Try eliminating all forms of caffeine, fried, processed and fatty foods for thirty days. Once you have overcome this challenge, you will no longer be subject to following your cravings. Instead, you will be ready to discover new, healthy foods and develop new eating habits that you will genuinely enjoy putting into practice.

As you cut down on bad habits, work to make improvements, too. Follow these basic guidelines:

- **Increase Choice:** Eat a wide variety of foods in a variety of amounts and combinations, but take care to still adhere to your recommended caloric allowance. By eating this way, you are more likely to consume all the vitamins, minerals and fatty acids that your body needs on a daily basis.

- **Eat Organic:** Avoid any vegetables, fruits and meats that are produced with pesticides, fertilizers, or other chemicals. Seek to eat fruits and vegetables that are as fresh as possible to ensure that you are getting the most vitamins and nutritional value (more on organic foods in the next chapter).

- **Eat Often:** It is best to eat small meals throughout the day. Enjoy a light meal as often as every four hours to keep your metabolism moving and your energy up.

- **Be Balanced:** Balance the consumption of lean animal and vegetable proteins with complex carbohydrates, healthy plant fats, and essential fatty acids (more on the definition of these food categories later in this chapter).

- **Drink Water:** Drink 8-10 glasses of purified water each day. Consuming a high quantity of healthy liquids keeps the bladder and kidneys operating regularly and enables the urethra to process fluids past the prostate gland.

Dietary Suggestions

Certain foods are highly recommended for maintaining a healthy prostate. In addition to following the basic guidelines listed above, look for these beneficial foods:

Seek out foods high in vitamin C, especially leafy green vegetables. Vegetables high in vitamin C are linked to a lower risk of developing prostate cancer. Additionally, leafy green vegetables (such as broccoli, kale and cabbage) contain quercetin and lycopene, which have been shown to have positive effects in cancer prevention.

Eat these vegetables on a regular basis:
- bell peppers
- broccoli
- brussel sprouts
- kohlrabi
- snow or snap peas
- cauliflower
- kale
- vegetable juices

Additionally, seek out these fruits:
- grapes
- grapefruit
- berries
- melons
- tomatoes

Addressing a Common Myth

A common myth claims that eating a can of tomatoes each week can prevent prostate cancer. Although this has been found to be untrue, tomatoes are still a good source of antioxidants, vitamin C and lycopene. No matter which vegetable you prefer, be sure to balance your consumption of that item by choosing to build a wide variety of other valuable fruits and vegetables into your diet.

Look for foods high in zinc. Foods rich in zinc (including cooked oysters, eggs, whole grains, nuts, fish, legumes, lima beans, mushrooms, pumpkin and sunflower seeds, sardines, soybeans, and poultry) have been shown to be beneficial for the prostate. Consuming lean beef and lamb cuts on occasion can also be a good source of zinc.

A Note on Protein

Many studies have been done regarding prostate health and a high protein intake, such as protein found in red meat. Some studies found that there was a higher risk for developing an enlarged prostate among men who consumed high quantities of red meat. This is often attributed to the possible rise in testosterone and hormone levels from red meat, which can potentially cause increased cell production in the prostate. However, others studies show that there is not a correlation between protein consumption and prostate cancer or BPH.

No matter what the latest study may say, it is best to be responsible about protein consumption by minimizing your consumption of red meat. Also, avoid meat that is high in fat and seek to supplement animal proteins with leaner, healthier sources of protein, such as beans or tofu. Consult your doctor if you are unsure about how much meat, or what kinds of protein, you should consume.

A Note on Supplements

Although there are many dietary and herbal supplements on the market that promise to help maintain prostate health, there is currently no concrete evidence that these are effective. Should you choose to take supplements, always make your doctor aware, and continue to practice healthy eating and exercise regularly. There is no substitute or short-cut to health. Making responsible choices about eating and exercise is the only way to be rewarded with health over the long-term, and will also help you to enjoy increased energy and vitality over the short-term.

Making a Change

Choosing to change your eating habits to ensure good health for years to come is a very important step, but getting started can be a challenge. Remember that big change doesn't happen overnight. Follow these basic guidelines to get you on the path to well-being:

Create a series of first steps based on your goals. Rather than focusing on a huge change, such as losing fifteen pounds, focus instead on losing small amounts of weight in increments. Plan steps on a week-by-week basis to help you reach this goal.

Begin keeping a food journal. Note the foods that you eat everyday. Pay close attention to when you slip up and overindulge. Did you have too much to eat on a particularly stressful day? Do you tend to drink more when socializing? Take note of tendencies like these so you can take steps to prevent them from happening again. Remember that occasional treats are okay, but overall you should maintain a healthful diet low in fat, in addition to keeping up with regular exercise.

Stress is often a major contributor to unhealthy habits. When we are stressed, we can get off track and eat poorly or neglect to exercise. Sources of stress can range from problems in the workplace to events that trigger strong feelings. Seek to reduce and manage stress as much as possible.

Managing Stress

Note what causes you stress. Keeping track of what events cause stress can help clue you in about the best ways to manage it. Ask yourself some key questions. Did an emotional event lead you to eat poorly? Is there a specific recurring situation that makes you irritable or frustrated, and causes you to neglect your health? Are you anxious about an upcoming event, such as moving or a new job? Keeping a journal and reviewing what upset your regular routine can help you anticipate these times when they happen again, and strengthen your resolve to resist temptation and maintain healthy habits. (Note: you might not discover right away the possible reasons for added pain or stress. Be patient. A positive attitude and strong will are extremely important.)

Once you figure out your possible stress triggers, watch out for those situations in order to avoid repeating them. Develop specific strategies for managing stress to help you get through the stressful event next time it occurs. Use helpful techniques to stay on track. These can include meditation as well as exercise.

Welcome help from others. The support of those who care about you can often mean the difference between success and failure. If you know a specific event or task causes you stress, enlist family or friends to help make the circumstances more manageable for you.

As you begin to implement changes in your life, be aware that psychological and physical stress can result. Don't let these factors steer you off course. Learn to help yourself through difficult times of stress through relaxation techniques such as meditation and yoga. If you find yourself with some free time, be sure to take advantage of it.

Remember that there are other ways to treat yourself besides eating fatty foods or consuming alcohol. You can instead indulge yourself by taking the time to enjoy a favorite activity or the company of friends. Being healthy on a regular basis, through stressful times as well as relaxing times, is key. Learning to care for yourself is imperative for your long-term health.

Lasting Change

Read as much as possible about prostate health. This will make you aware of symptoms of an enlarged prostate so that you know when to seek out a doctor's opinion (remember, a condition like BPH is one that can worsen over time). Educating yourself about what to expect is a great way to empower yourself. Should you or someone you care about face any specific prostate-related health issues, you will be prepared and ready to make informed decisions about treatment options.

Reaching Out to Others

Be sure to remember that those around you are an important component of a healthy, meaningful life. Work on maintaining strong relationships with those closest to you. It is vital that you let your friends and family member know you need their support in order to maintain healthy habits over time. Those who are nearest to you will help provide a source of strength as well as motivation to stay healthy.

If family or friends want to know more about how they can help, you can even give them a copy of this book. Explain that the recipes are low-fat and highly beneficial for maintaining a healthy prostate. If you cook as a family, make family members aware that it would mean a great deal if these meals could be incorporated into the weekly family meal plan. Let friends know that you need to watch your diet and make responsible food choices when you dine together. You can even try cooking together. Divide tasks (such as food preparation, cooking, and cleaning up) among friends or family members. The reward will be more than just sharing a memorable meal; you will all learn how to cook for health, as well.

Chapter 3

Dietary Suggestions for a Healthy Lifestyle

No matter what your health problems, eating healthy foods should be a priority. You need to be responsible for your own health; don't expect anyone to keep you in line. As a matter of fact, many people will offer you foods that are not good for you. It is ultimately up to you to stay on track with your eating goals and say, "no thank you." Always pay attention to your nutrition plan and do everything in your power to stay as close to it as possible.

Keep in mind that you may slip up—this is understandable. Eating habits are difficult to change and are often rooted in years of cultural and family habits. Expecting a quick change is not realistic. Patience and a strong will to change over time are a must.

Healthy eating is not about eating everything you like. It is about giving your body what it needs and what agrees with it. It is about eating the right amount of calories per day considering your daily activities. Eating healthy is also about meal rituals. That means having regular meals at the same times every day. Three to four meals a day is recommended. This includes a snack in the afternoon, which is important to keep your blood sugar level stable if you have a late dinner. It is ultimately up to you to decide what works best for your body and how to spread your meals throughout your day. Remember to appropriately divide your daily calories.

Eating should be a pleasant experience, too. Fresh fruits and vegetables and lean meats, when eaten plain or in a delicious recipe, can brighten your day. You will feel much better knowing that your food choices are enriching your life and possibly helping to reduce painful symptoms. By employing new habits, you will eventually see the fruits of your labor in an improved overall well-being.

Eating Organic

Everyone knows that eating foods that are free of pesticides, chemicals, antibiotics, colorings, or hormones is better for you. If you are not financially strained, make an effort to shop organic at your local farmers' market, growers, and stores. If budget is an issue, do not stress about it. Sometimes we have to make practical decisions and, understandably, eating organic may not always be a priority. Also, keep in mind that due to very strict regulations, many farmers and growers are not able to obtain the organic label but are still producing foods that are free of pesticides, chemicals, antibiotics, and hormones, and are of excellent quality. All you need to do is find those products in your local stores and read their labels carefully.

Below are some buying tips for eating healthy while on a budget:

When buying dry, canned, or frozen products you should make sure to buy organic. They are not much more expensive and are much healthier for you. While you should not be eating such products on a regular basis, they can be helpful during the winter months, when a variety of vegetables and fruits are not available. Also, if you cook for yourself and feel physically exhausted, you might opt for the dry, canned or frozen product.

Reduce your individual portions, particularly with meat products. You can stretch your dollars while you shrink your waistline. Portion sizes at your local store are often larger than what you really need to eat. For example, a chicken breast often weighs 8 ounces when you should only be eating about 4 ounces.

Support your local farmers and growers. The more distance the food travels from farm to table, the greater the cost. Join a food co-op. Co-ops purchase food in bulk and often carry organic items. If there isn't one in your town, consider starting one with family and friends.

Share your knowledge. If you have discovered healthy organic or non-organic foods from a reputable supplier, pass the news on via an e-mail to friends. They will appreciate it immensely and you will help promote such suppliers, which eventually will be in a better position to lower prices based on demand.

Eating Out

Preferably, you should eat out no more than twice a week. Keep that time for the weekend with family and friends. Too many restaurants use commercially packaged, high-sodium food and unhealthy fats, which are detrimental to your health. It is extremely important that you pay attention to the type of foods you choose when going out.

In a restaurant, do not hesitate to question the waiter about the ingredients in a particular dish. Let him or her know you are on a specific diet and looking for nutrient-rich dishes that are also low in fat. More and more chefs are willing to accommodate their clients today because they know it is important for the survival of the restaurant. There is also an increased demand for healthier choices, and the industry is paying attention. Choosing a restaurant that caters to foods closer to your diet (such as Italian, Mediterranean, or vegetarian restaurants) is also wise—chances are you will find more food that you can enjoy there in the first place.

Quick Tips for Ordering at a Restaurant

- Order steamed vegetables with olive oil or lemon on the side.
- Brown rice is also safe.
- Ask for your dish to be prepared with a bit of olive oil, canola oil, or grape seed oil instead of butter. Ask for olive oil and vinegar on the side for your salad dressing or bring your own dressing.
- Half a baked potato is safe as long as it is without toppings and butter (you can always drizzle a little olive oil over it yourself).
- Stay away from unhealthy carbohydrates and ask to substitute steamed vegetables instead. Avoid most desserts except fresh fruits. It is best to save your sweet tooth for homemade, healthier goodies that feature abundant amounts of fresh fruit.
- Don't blindly eat what is served to you—pay attention to the type of food and the amount of food, and try to figure out the total calories. Put that into perspective with your meal allowance.

When visiting with family or friends, make them aware of your health situation a few days before the visit. If they already know, just give them a quick phone call to remind them, as many people have a very active lifestyle and may easily forget. Be very diligent and carefully choose what you eat. If needed, ask the host if he or she made the food from scratch, what is in it, or if it is store bought food. Remember: when in doubt, do not eat it. If you are not sure of the situation, you can always eat before you go to an event. If you know that the food the host prepares will not agree with you, ask if you can bring your own food. No one should get upset; after all it is about making sure everyone enjoys the party!

While traveling, keep the same attitude that you have when you are eating out close to home. Be even more vigilant. It is best to bring your own food, but sometimes this is not possible (such as when traveling by airplane). When booking your flight, most airlines will gladly reserve a low-fat meal for you. Vegetarian meals may also be a good choice, but use caution as they are often based on cheese and carbohydrates. Ask specifically what foods are included in the meals. At the airport, look for food that is freshly prepared in front of you and as close as possible to your nutritional plan. Take with you enough snack foods to last you a day or two in case of schedule delays. Nuts, raisins, and dates are easy to carry. You will be able to find bottles of water, milk, or juice in most places.

When traveling abroad, be even more careful than you would be at home. Foods are not prepared the same way and many unknown ingredients may be a real problem to your health. Stick with plain grilled, steamed, broiled, or baked main courses with rice, potatoes, or steamed vegetables as side dishes. If you have no choice, pick the healthiest option and eat what you know is safe for you. Be careful with raw foods, as sanitation may not be as thorough as at home. Always ask for a bottle of water to be opened in front of you. Don't miss the opportunity to go to a local market and purchase some fresh fruits, vegetables, and healthy snacks such as almonds, walnuts, hazelnuts, dates, or whatever you may be able to keep in your hotel room.

Don't forget to wash the vegetables and fruits with a bottle of water mixed with a little vinegar. This will help kill bacteria not visible to the eye. If you have a refrigerator in the room, stock it with milk, yogurt, or cheese to provide you with low-fat sources of calcium and protein. Read all food labels carefully. If you don't understand the language, this may be a problem. See if the concierge or a person speaking your language at the hotel can assist you. Be on your guard at all times. If you take supplements or specific medications, make sure you have enough for your trip, plus a week's worth as back-up.

Remember, whether you have to travel or dine out, there is always a way to eat healthy. Knowing as much as you can about eating well will help you make good choices. Cooking for yourself at home is one of the best ways to learn. Use the recipes in the next section to get started. Cook as often as you can, and enjoy experimenting based on what you like, as well as what is healthiest for you. Take care to consume a wide variety of fresh fruits and vegetables as well as good sources of lean protein. Use what you learn about nutrition, as well as about your own personal tastes, to make responsible— and delicious—food choices. Smart choices and good habits will empower you to enjoy each day, knowing that you are ensuring your long-term health.

Chapter 4

The Recipes

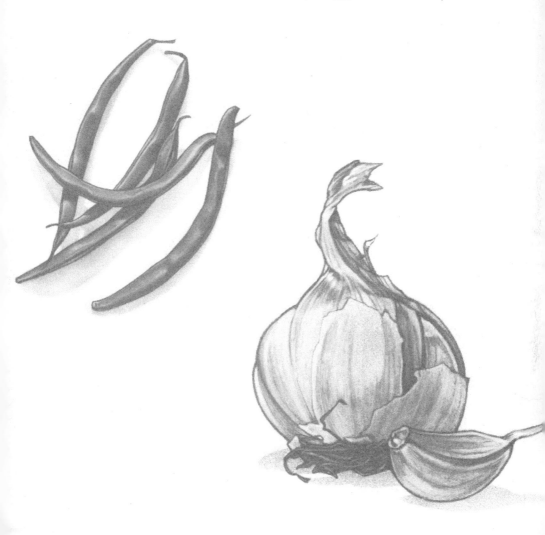

Breakfast

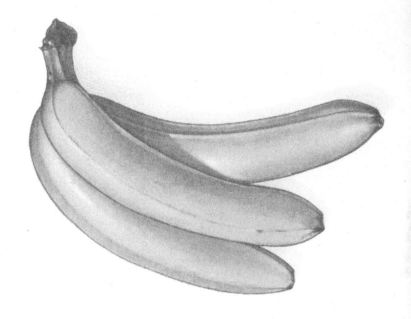

Cream of Millet

serves 1

ingredients

¾ cup to 1 cup low-fat milk
(cow's, rice, soy, or nut)
1 teaspoon pumpkin pie spice (optional)
Small pinch of salt
¼ cup pearl millet
2 teaspoons slivered almonds
2 teaspoons maple syrup
½ peach, peeled and diced
1 teaspoon flaxseed oil

✓ *If you use less cooking liquid than prescribed here, the grain will be fluffier and crunchier. Using more liquid will create moister, softer texture. It is all about personal preferences, so experiment and find the texture you like.*

You may substitute flaxseed oil with 1 teaspoon ground flaxseeds.

Feel free to exchange the peach for apricot, apple, mango, or berries.

cooking instructions

Warm up the milk, the spice, (if using), and salt over medium heat. Wash the millet a couple of times and drain well. Place the millet in a pan. Add the almonds and the warmed spiced milk. Reduce heat and simmer for 20 minutes or until all the liquid is absorbed.

Transfer to a serving bowl and mix in the maple syrup. Top with the peach, drizzle flaxseed oil, and serve immediately.

Salmon and Asparagus Omelet

serves 4

ingredients

2 teaspoons canola oil
½ small onion, diced
1 garlic clove, minced
8 asparagus spears, cooked
1 teaspoon lemon juice
8 eggs
1 tablespoon low-fat milk
1 teaspoon minced fresh chives

1 teaspoon minced fresh dill
2 tablespoons minced fresh parsley
4 slices smoked salmon, cut into strips
(about 4 ounces)
Salt and pepper to taste

cooking instructions

Heat the oil in a nonstick pan over medium heat. Add the onion and sauté until translucent. Add the garlic, asparagus and lemon juice, and sauté for 2 minutes. Spread the vegetables evenly on the bottom of the pan.

In a bowl, beat the eggs, milk, and herbs, and season with salt and pepper. Add the egg mixture to the vegetables in the pan and let the eggs set, about 1½ minutes. Add the smoked salmon, reduce heat, and continue to cook for 2 to 3 minutes. Fold the omelet over in half, cook for 1 more minute, and serve immediately.

Provençal Omelet

serves 4

ingredients

1 large tomato
2 teaspoons olive oil
½ small onion, diced
3 garlic cloves, minced
1 large bell pepper, ribs removed, seeded, and diced

⅔ cup cooked spinach, chopped
2 tablespoons minced fresh salad herbs
8 eggs
1 tablespoon low-fat milk
Salt and pepper to taste

cooking instructions

Make a small X incision at the top and bottom of the tomato. Blanch the tomato for 20 seconds. Place in ice-cold water to stop the cooking process. Peel, seed, and dice the tomato.

Heat the oil in a nonstick pan over medium heat. Add the onions and sauté until translucent. Add the garlic and bell pepper, and cook for 3 minutes. Add the diced tomato and sauté briefly. Add the spinach and salad herbs, and season with salt and pepper. Spread the vegetables evenly over the bottom of the pan.

In a bowl, beat the eggs and milk, then season. Add the egg mixture to the vegetables and let the eggs set. Reduce heat and continue to cook for 2 to 3 minutes. Fold the omelet in half, cook for 1 more minute, and serve immediately.

Muesli with Peach and Almonds

serves 1

✔ *Option:*
Add 1 tablespoon
of flaxseeds

ingredients

½ cup Muesli cereal
½ cup low-fat yogurt
2 teaspoons almonds, slivered or sliced
1 small peach
Low-fat milk

cooking instructions

In a bowl mix the cereal with the yogurt. Thin out with a little milk. Top with the peaches and almonds, then serve immediately.

Kasha with Apples and Cinnamon

serves 1

✓ *You may serve with more milk, take over if desired.*

ingredients

⅔ cup low-fat milk
(cow's, rice, soy, or nut)
2 tablespoons buckwheat groats
¼ teaspoon cinnamon
Pinch of salt
½ apple, diced

1 tablespoon raisins
1 teaspoon freshly ground
flaxseed
1 tablespoon honey

cooking instructions

In a saucepan, bring the milk to boil. Add the buckwheat groats, cinnamon, and salt. Mix and bring to boil. Reduce heat and simmer for 10 to 12 minutes.

Transfer to a serving bowl. Top with the diced apple, raisins, and flaxseeds. Drizzle honey and serve immediately.

Muesli with Berries

serves 1

ingredients

½ cup muesli cereal
½ cup low-fat plain yogurt
2 teaspoons almonds
2 ounces berries (about ⅖ cup)
Low-fat milk (to thin out, if desired)

cooking instructions

In a bowl, mix the cereal with the yogurt. If desired, thin out with a little milk. Top with the berries and raisins, then serve immediately.

Oat Bran–Flax Muffin

serves 12

ingredients

1 cup unbleached all-purpose flour
½ cup oat bran flour
½ cup flaxseed meal
½ cup brown sugar
1½ teaspoons baking soda
1 teaspoon baking powder
¼ teaspoon salt
1½ tablespoons ground cinnamon
1 teaspoon ground ginger
1¼ cup shredded peeled carrots

2 medium apples, peeled, cored, and finely diced
¾ cup walnuts, chopped
¾ cup dried berries and raisins blend (about equal amount of each)
¼ cup canola oil
1 teaspoon vanilla extract
2 eggs, mixed
½ cup low-fat milk

✔ *Careful, this recipe can act as a laxative. It is advisable to eat only one muffin per day. Muffins can be frozen once individually wrapped in cellophane and then placed in a freezer bag. For best results, defrost at room temperature for 1 hour.*

cooking instructions

Preheat the oven to 350°F.

In a bowl, blend the flours, flaxseed meal, brown sugar, baking soda, baking powder, salt, cinnamon, and ginger. Mix in the carrots, apples, walnuts, and berry-raisin blend. Add the oil, vanilla, eggs, and milk, and mix until incorporated. Grease the muffin tin with canola oil. Divide mix among the 12 cups of a muffin tin and bake between 20 to 25 minutes.

Rye Bread with Cream Cheese and Salmon

serves 1

✔ *Option: You may mix in a bit of freshly minced dill and some lemon juice into the cream cheese before spreading over the bread.*

ingredients

1½ tablespoons low-fat cream cheese
1 slice rye bread
1 slice smoked salmon (about ¾ ounces)
Lemon juice

cooking instructions

Spread the cream cheese over the bread. Add the smoked salmon, sprinkle a little lemon juice, and serve immediately.

Wheat Bran Flakes with Berries and Raisins

serves 1

ingredients

1 cup wheat bran flakes
½ cup low-fat milk
¼ cup mixed fresh berries
1 tablespoon raisins
1 teaspoon flaxseeds

cooking instructions

In a bowl, mix the cereal with the milk. Top with the berries, raisins, and flaxseeds, and serve immediately.

Buckwheat Crêpes with Cottage Cheese and Berries

serves 10

ingredients

½ cup all-purpose flour
½ cup buckwheat flour
2 eggs
1 tablespoon maple syrup
2 tablespoons grapeseed oil, plus more for the pan, or 2 tablespoons unsalted butter, melted

10 tablespoons maple syrup, plus 1 tablespoon for batter
1 teaspoon vanilla extract
Pinch salt
1 cup low-fat milk
8 ounces low-fat cottage cheese
2 cups fresh berries

cooking instructions

Place the flours in a bowl. Blend in the eggs, the 2 tablespoons grapeseed oil, 1 tablespoon of the maple syrup, the vanilla, and salt. Slowly, whisk in the milk. Let the batter rest for 30 minutes. Before using, add a little water to thin out.

Heat a medium-sized nonstick pan or crêpe pan over medium heat. Soak a small piece of a paper towel with 1 teaspoon grapeseed oil and swirl the greased towel quickly over the pan. Add enough batter to cover the entire bottom and swirl. Cook until golden brown and turn over. Cook the second side until golden brown as well. Repeat this process until all the crêpe batter is used.

Fill each crêpe with about ¾ ounce (about 1½ tablespoons) low-fat cottage cheese and roll up. Top with 3 tablespoons berries (there will be some left when done) and 1 tablespoon maple syrup each.

Breakfast Smoothie

serves 2

✓ *This breakfast smoothie also makes a perfect snack during the day.*

ingredients

4 ounces pure pomegranate juice, no sugar added
1 cup mixed berries
1 small banana
½ cup apple juice, no sugar added
1 tablespoon flaxseeds
Ice cubes

cooking instructions

Place all the ingredients in a blender and fill with ice. Puree on high speed until smooth. Divide between two tall glasses and serve immediately with a straw.

All-Bran with Apples and Cinnamon

serves 1

✓ *You may substitute low-fat milk with low-fat soy milk, low-fat rice milk, or low-fat almond milk.*

ingredients

1 cup all bran flakes
½ cup low-fat milk
¼ cup apples
1 tablespoon raisins
1 teaspoon freshly ground flaxseeds
Cinnamon to taste (optional)

cooking instructions

In a bowl mix the cereal with the milk. Top with the apples, raisins, and flaxseeds. Sprinkle with cinnamon and serve immediately.

Oatmeal with Kiwi and Banana

serves 1

✓ *Option:*
Add 1 teaspoon
flaxseed

ingredients

½ cup to ¾ cup oatmeal
1 cup to 1½ cups low-fat milk, hot
1 teaspoon almonds
1 kiwi, diced
½ banana, diced

cooking instructions

Mix the oatmeal with the hot milk until the liquid is incorporated. Add in the almonds, kiwi, banana, and serve immediately.

French Toast with Orange Slices

serves 4

✓ *For variety you may flavor with cinnamon and nutmeg.*

ingredients

3 eggs
⅔ cup low-fat milk
1½ teaspoon orange extract
Pinch salt
8 slices whole wheat bread
4 tablespoons maple syrup
2 oranges, peeled and sliced
Vegetable oil

cooking instructions

Beat together the eggs, milk, orange extract, and salt. Dip the bread slices in the mixture. Soak them well.

Preheat two large skillets or a griddle with a little vegetable oil. Add the bread slices and brown on both sides. Serve immediately with maple syrup and orange slices.

Soups & Salads

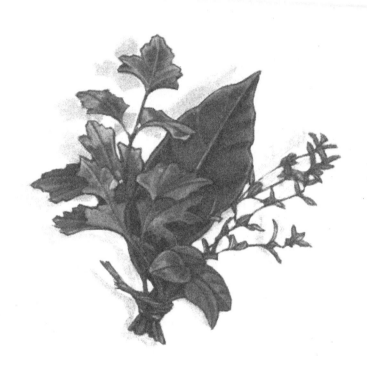

Broccoli Soup

serves 4

ingredients

2 teaspoons grapeseed oil
1 small onion, diced (about 4 ounces)
4 large broccoli heads, chopped (about 2 pounds)
1 garlic clove, minced
3 cups chicken or vegetable stock (low-fat and low-sodium)
1 bouquet garni
1 cup low-fat milk
2 to 3 tablespoons cornstarch mixed with a little water
Salt and pepper to taste

cooking instructions

Heat the oil in a large pan over high heat. Add the onion and sauté
until translucent. Add ¾ of the broccoli, garlic, stock, and bouquet garni,
then bring to a boil. Reduce heat and simmer until the broccoli is very
tender. Remove the bouquet garni and puree with a hand blender. Add
the milk and bring back to a boil. Thicken with arrowroot/cornstarch
water mixture, a little at a time, until you reach the desired consistency.
Add the remaining broccoli and bring to a boil. Cook until tender, adjust
seasonings, and serve immediately.

Lentil Soup with Ground Turkey

serves 4

ingredients

3 teaspoons canola oil
1 large onion, diced small
(about 8 ounces)
1 large carrot, diced small
(about 4 ounces)
2 large celery stalks, diced small
(about 4 ounces)
2 garlic cloves, minced

6 cups chicken stock
(low-fat and low-sodium)
3 cups dried lentils
1 bouquet garni
8 ounces ground turkey
Salt and pepper to taste

cooking instructions

Heat 2 teaspoons of oil in a large pan over high heat. Add the onion and sauté until translucent. Add the carrot, celery, and garlic, then cook for 2 minutes. Add the stock, lentils, and bouquet garni, then bring to a boil. Reduce heat, cover, and simmer for 35 minutes. Skim the surface as needed. Continue to simmer uncovered for 10 minutes in order to thicken the soup. Remove the bouquet garni. Heat 1 teaspoon of oil in a medium pan over high heat. Add the ground turkey and sauté until cooked through (about 3 to 4 minutes). Strain and discard any fat. Add the meat to the prepared lentils and bring to a boil. Adjust seasonings and serve immediately.

If the soup turns out too thick, adjust with stock. If the soup is too thin, reduce the liquid more or mash a little bit of the lentils and return mixture to the pan.

Cod and Corn Chowder

serves 4

ingredients

2 teaspoons grapeseed oil
1 medium onion, diced
(about 6 ounces)
1 medium carrot, diced
(about 3 ounces)
1 large celery stalk, diced
(about 2 ounces)
2 medium potatoes, peeled and
diced (about 12 ounces)

2 cups vegetable stock
(low-fat and low-sodium)
Corn kernels from 2 corn ears
1 cup low-fat milk
1 pound cod fish fillets, diced
2 tablespoons freshly minced
parsley
Salt and pepper to taste

cooking instructions

Heat the oil in a saucepan over high heat. Add the onion and sauté until translucent. Add the carrot, celery, potatoes, and stock, then bring to a boil. Reduce heat and simmer for 15 minutes. Mash the potato with a fork and continue to reduce until you obtain a creamy texture. Add the corn, milk, fish, and parsley, then bring to a boil. Continue to simmer for another 5 minutes. Adjust seasoning and serve immediately.

Chickpea, Tomato, and Rice Soup

serves 4

ingredients

1 teaspoon olive oil
1 small onion, diced (about 4 ounces)
1 (8 oz.) can chopped Italian plum tomatoes
½ cup brown rice
12 ounces cooked chickpeas
3 garlic cloves, minced

5 cups chicken stock
½ teaspoon fresh rosemary, minced
2 tablespoons fresh parsley, chopped
Salt and pepper to taste

cooking instructions

Heat the oil in a large pan over high heat. Add the onion and sauté until translucent. Add the garlic, tomatoes, and rosemary, then cook until the juices are evaporated. Add the rice and stock, then bring to boil. Reduce heat, cover, and simmer for 25 minutes. Add the chickpeas and continue to cook for 5 minutes, or until the rice is cooked through. Add the parsley, season to taste, and serve immediately.

Vegetable Soup

serves 6

ingredients

2 small fresh tomatoes
(about 6 ounces)
2 teaspoons canola oil
1 large onion, diced
(about 8 ounces)
2 large celery stalks, diced
(about 4 ounces)
1 small leek, chopped
(about 4 ounces)
1 large carrot, diced
(about 4 ounces)
1 medium red bell pepper,
seeded, ribs removed, and diced
(about 6 ounces)

1 large turnip, diced
(about 6 ounces)
2 garlic cloves, minced
6 cups vegetable or chicken stock
(low-fat and low-sodium)
1 bouquet garni
1 bunch spinach, chopped
2 tablespoons freshly minced
parsley
Salt and pepper to taste

✓ *You can easily double this recipe and use it for a variety of meals or freeze portions. Add brown rice, diced chicken, diced turkey, meatballs (made from ground turkey, venison, or buffalo), fish pieces, shellfish, or tofu.*

To make a puree of vegetables: Cook the vegetables until they start to fall apart and transfer to a food mill.

cooking instructions

Make a small X incision at the top and bottom of the tomatoes. Blanch the tomatoes for 20 seconds. Remove and place in ice-cold water to stop the cooking process. Peel, seed, and dice the tomatoes.

Heat the oil in a large pan over medium-high heat. Add the onion and sauté until translucent. Add the celery, leek, carrot, and bell pepper, and sauté for about 1 minute. Add the turnip, garlic, stock, and bouquet garni, and bring to a boil. Reduce heat and simmer until the vegetables are almost cooked through, but still a bit crunchy. Add the tomatoes and spinach, and simmer for 1 minute. Finish with the parsley and season with salt and pepper.

Gazpacho

serves 12

ingredients

4 slices whole wheat bread
½ cup olive oil
7 large tomatoes, chopped
(about 2 ½ pounds)
2 medium cucumbers, chopped
(about 1 pound)
1 large onion, chopped
(about 8 ounces)
1 medium red or orange bell
pepper, seeded, ribs removed,
and chopped (about 6 ounces)
6 garlic cloves, chopped

2 cups tomato juice
¼ cup red wine vinegar
2 tablespoons chopped fresh basil
1 tablespoon chopped fresh
tarragon
Dash ground cumin
Dash Tabasco® sauce
1 lemon, juiced
Salt and cayenne pepper to taste

cooking instructions

Soak the bread in approximately ¼ cup cold water for 5 minutes.

In a blender, puree all the ingredients until smooth. Season with salt and cayenne pepper. Refrigerate and serve cold.

Fish Soup

serves 8

> ✔ *The following fish work best for this soup: cod, bream, eel, haddock, hake, mackerel, monkfish, perch, red snapper, or white fish. Remember, the total calories will vary depending on the fish selected.*

ingredients

2 medium tomatoes
(about 8 ounces)
2 teaspoons olive oil
1 large onion, finely diced
(about 8 ounces)
1 large carrot, finely diced
(about 4 ounces)
5 garlic cloves, minced
6 ounces Chardonnay
(with lemon and butter tones)
6 cups fish stock (low-sodium)
1 bouquet garni
¼ cup minced fresh parsley

2 long and wide strips orange zest
4 saffron threads
1 teaspoon fennel seeds
2 large potatoes, peeled and
quartered (about 1 pound)
4 pounds various fish (see note
above)
2 tablespoons freshly chopped
basil
Salt and pepper to taste

cooking instructions

Make a small X incision at the tops and bottoms of the tomatoes. Blanch for 20 seconds. Remove and place the tomatoes in ice-cold water to stop the cooking process. Peel, seed, and dice the tomatoes. Set aside.

Heat the oil in a large deep pan over high heat. Add the onion and sauté until translucent. Add the carrots and garlic, then sauté for 2 minutes. Add the wine and reduce by half. Add the stock, bouquet garni, tomatoes, parsley, orange zest, saffron, fennel seeds, and potatoes, then bring to a boil. Reduce heat and simmer for 10 minutes. Add the fish and basil, then simmer for another 10 minutes. Check the potatoes and fish. If done, remove the bouquet garni and orange zest. Skim the surface of any foam that formed, season with salt and pepper, and serve immediately.

Mushroom and Barley Soup

serves 4

ingredients

2 teaspoons grapeseed oil

⅓ cup barley (about 2 ounces)

1 small onion, diced
(about 4 ounces)

1 large carrot, diced
(about 4 ounces)

1 small turnip, diced
(about 4 ounces)

4 cups chicken or vegetable stock
(low-fat and low-sodium)

1 bouquet garni

8 ounces mushrooms, peeled and
diced

1 cup low-fat milk

2 tablespoons minced parsley

Salt and pepper to taste

cooking instructions

Cook the barley according to package directions. Drain and set aside.

Heat the oil in a pan over high heat. Add the onion, carrot, and turnip,
then sauté for 2 minutes. Add the stock and bouquet garni, then bring to
a boil. Reduce heat and simmer until the vegetables are barely tender. Add
the mushrooms, drained barley, and milk, then bring to a simmer. Continue
to cook for 3 to 5 minutes. Add parsley, adjust seasonings, and serve
immediately.

Smoked Salmon, Potato, and Watercress Salad

serves 4

ingredients

12 ounces smoked salmon, diced
3 cooked potatoes, sliced (about 1 pound)
1 bunch watercress
1 cup cooked broccoli
1 hardboiled egg, chopped (or 2 egg whites for less cholesterol)

2 tablespoons white wine vinegar
4 tablespoons olive oil
1 teaspoon Dijon mustard
1 tablespoon minced shallots
2 tablespoons minced salad herb
Salt and pepper to taste

cooking instructions

Mix the vinegar, mustard, and shallots in a bowl. Whisk in the olive oil, 1 tablespoon of minced herbs, and season to taste.

Mix half of the dressing with the potatoes. Mix the remaining dressing with the watercress. Divide the watercress among four plates. Top with the potatoes, broccoli, and salmon. Sprinkle with the chopped egg, remaining minced herbs, and serve immediately.

Salmon and Asparagus Salad

serves 4

ingredients

5 ounces salad greens
16 asparagus stalks
1 large bulb fennel, sliced thinly
(about 12 ounces)
4 four-ounce salmon fillets
1 teaspoon Dijon mustard
2 tablespoons orange juice

1 teaspoon orange zest
4 tablespoons olive oil
1 tablespoon salad herbs, minced
1 orange, peeled and sliced
Salt and pepper to taste

cooking instructions

In a bowl mix the mustard, juice, oil, zest, herbs, and season to taste.

Preheat a steamer. Trim the asparagus and place them in the steamer basket. Cook until barely tender. Transfer the asparagus to a platter and let cool.

Season the salmon fillets and add to the steamer basket. Top with the fennel slices and steam until cooked through, about 10 to 12 minutes. Time may vary based on the thickness of the fillets.

Mix the dressing with the greens. Divide equally among four plates. Top with the fillets, fennel, asparagus, orange slices, and serve immediately.

Chicken Salad with Fruit

serves 4

ingredients

5 ounces fresh mixed greens
12 ounces cooked chicken breasts
(without skin), diced
1 avocado, diced
1 large apple, diced
(about 6 ounces)
1 orange, peeled and wedged
(about 6 ounces)
2 kiwis, peeled and sliced
(about 6 ounces)

4 teaspoons pumpkin seeds
2 tablespoons olive oil
2 tablespoons lemon juice
1 tablespoon fresh salad herbs
Large pinch of each curry
and ginger
4 ounces reduced fat goat cheese,
sliced
Salt and pepper to taste

cooking instructions

In a bowl mix the oil, lemon, and herbs. Blend in the curry, ginger, and season to taste.

In a bowl mix the greens with 2/3 of the prepared dressing. Equally divide the greens among four plates. Top with the chicken, fruit, avocado, pumpkin seeds, and goat cheese. Drizzle the remaining dressing and serve immediately.

White Beans and Tuna Salad

serves 6

ingredients

2 cups cooked white beans
8 ounces cooked tuna
2 scallions, chopped
2 tomatoes; peeled, seeded, and
diced (about 12 ounces)
1 medium yellow bell pepper; cut
in half, seeded, and ribs removed
(about 6 ounces)

1 tablespoon freshly minced
parsley
1 tablespoon freshly minced
tarragon
2 tablespoons lemon juice
4 tablespoons olive oil
Salt and pepper to taste

cooking instructions

Preheat the broiler. Place the bell pepper halves, opening down, on a cookie sheet. Broil until the skin is completely browned. Place in a brown bag, seal, and let stand for 10 minutes. Remove the bell pepper skin and dice.

Place the beans, tuna, scallions, and parsley in a bowl. Mix with half the lemon juice and half the olive oil. Season with pepper and salt. Transfer to an elongated platter. Spread the tomatoes, bell pepper pieces and adjust seasonings. Sprinkle with the remaining lemon juice and olive oil before serving.

Artichoke and Fava Bean Salad

serves 4

> ✔ *If fava beans are unavailable, use butter beans, broad beans, Windsor beans, or lima beans.*

ingredients

For the vinaigrette:
2 shallots, minced
1 large garlic clove, minced
1 teaspoon Dijon mustard
4 tablespoons balsamic vinegar
6 tablespoons olive oil
2 tablespoons flaxseed oil (or olive oil, if flaxseed oil unavailable)
3 tablespoons salad herbs
Salt and pepper to taste

For the salad:
4 ounces Boston lettuce
8 ounces cooked fava beans
1 cup cooked artichoke hearts
8 cherry tomatoes
4 ounces feta cheese, cut into 1-inch cubes
4 teaspoons slivered almonds

cooking instructions

For the vinaigrette: In a bowl, mix the shallots, garlic, mustard, and vinegar. Slowly whisk in the oils. Add the herbs and season with salt and pepper.

For the salad: Line a serving platter with the lettuce. Spread the fava beans, artichokes hearts, and tomatoes on top of the lettuce. Drizzle with the vinaigrette. Add the feta cheese and almonds, and serve immediately.

Belgium Endives with Gorgonzola

serves 4

ingredients

6 Belgium endives (about 1 pound)
¼ cup walnuts, chopped
2 ounces Gorgonzola
2 tablespoons walnut oil
1 tablespoon red wine vinegar

1 tablespoon low-fat milk
mixed with a dash of mashed
Gorgonzola
1 tablespoon fresh salad herbs,
chopped
Salt and pepper to taste

cooking instructions

Mix the oil, vinegar, and milk mixture. Add herbs and season to taste.

Slice the endives. Discard the trunk of each endive. Wash and dry the endives with a salad spinner. Transfer to a bowl and mix with the dressing. Add the walnuts and the crumbled remaining Gorgonzola. Toss lightly and serve immediately.

Carrot and Apple Salad

serves 4

ingredients

For the vinaigrette:
1 large garlic clove, minced
1 teaspoon Dijon mustard
2 tablespoons lemon juice
2 tablespoons canola oil
2 tablespoons flaxseed oil
(or canola oil, if flaxseed oil
unavailable)
1 tablespoon minced fresh parsley
Salt and pepper to taste

For the salad:
4 large carrots (about 1 pound)
1 large apple (about 6 ounces)
4 teaspoons walnuts

cooking instructions

For the vinaigrette: In a bowl, mix the garlic, mustard, and lemon juice. Blend in the oils. Add the parsley, and season with salt and pepper.

For the salad: Peel and shred the carrots, then immediately mix with the vinaigrette. Peel, core, and shred the apples, then immediately add to the carrots. Blend well and adjust seasonings. Add the walnuts and serve immediately.

Chef Marie Nicoise Salad

serves 4

ingredients

For the dressing:
1 shallot, minced
1 garlic clove, minced
1 teaspoon Dijon mustard
2 tablespoons wine vinegar
4 tablespoons olive oil
2 tablespoons walnut oil
2 tablespoons salad herbs
2 anchovy fillets
Pepper
Salt to taste

For the salad:
4 eggs
5 ounces mixed greens
2 large tomatoes, seeded and diced
2 cooked medium potatoes, sliced
1 orange bell pepper, seeded, ribs removed, and julienned
1 small cucumber, peeled and sliced
4 ounces cooked green beans, cut in half
6 ounces tuna, canned in water, strained
1 tablespoon salad herbs
2 ounces small Niçoise black olives
Salt to taste

cooking instructions

For the dressing: In a bowl, mix the shallot, garlic, mustard, vinegar, oils, salad herbs, anchovy fillets, and a pinch of pepper. Puree with a hand blender. If too thick, add a little water to thin out. Taste and adjust seasonings.

For the salad: Place the eggs in a pan, cover with cold water, add 2 teaspoons salt, and bring to a boil over medium heat. Reduce heat and simmer for 10 minutes. Remove the eggs and place them in cold water. Peel, quarter, and set aside.

In a large bowl, mix the mixed greens with ¾ of the dressing. Transfer to a serving platter. Add the tomatoes, potatoes, bell pepper, cucumber, and green beans. Top with the tuna, eggs, and olives, then sprinkle the remaining herbs. Drizzle the remaining dressing and serve immediately.

Grapefruit and Crabmeat Salad

serves 2

ingredients

1 large pink grapefruit
(about 16 ounces grapefruit)
8 ounces crabmeat portions,
excess water removed
2 tablespoons low-fat canola
mayonnaise

1 cup lettuce, shredded
1 tablespoon freshly minced
cilantro
Chili powder to taste
Salt and pepper to taste

cooking instructions

Place the crabmeat in a bowl.

Cut the grapefruit in half. Insert a thin knife all around the skin to loosen up the flesh. Separate the flesh from the skin and place it on a cutting board. Dice the flesh small and transfer to the crabmeat bowl. Add mayonnaise, chili powder, cilantro, and season to taste. Cover with plastic wrap and refrigerate for half an hour.

Equally divide the lettuce in two plates and top with the prepared grapefruit crabmeat salad.

Tomato and Basil Salad

serves 4

ingredients

6 to 8 fresh basil leaves
6 large tomatoes (about 2 pounds)
1 shallot, minced
1 large garlic clove, minced
2 tablespoons balsamic vinegar
(preferably aged)

3 tablespoons olive oil
1 tablespoon flaxseed oil (or olive
oil, if flaxseed oil unavailable)
1 tablespoon minced fresh parsley
Salt and pepper to taste

cooking instructions

Mince half the basil leaves and shred the remaining half.

Cut off each end of the tomatoes and discard. Slice the tomatoes and spread them on a plate. Sprinkle them with a little salt and set aside for 20 minutes.

In a bowl, mix the shallot, garlic, and vinegar, then whisk in the oils. Add the minced basil and parsley, then season with salt and pepper.

Transfer the tomatoes to serving platter. Sprinkle the shredded basil, pour over the dressing, and serve immediately.

Quinoa and Apricot Salad

serves 4

✔ *Note: for a more flavorful dish, substitute stock for the water in this recipe.*

ingredients

1 cup quinoa
2 teaspoons olive oil
1 small red onion, diced
(about 4 ounces)
2 mushrooms, diced
(about 2 ounces)
1 tablespoon freshly minced
ginger root
1 small green jalapeño, minced
1 teaspoon turmeric

1 teaspoon ground coriander
¼ teaspoon ground cinnamon
1 lemon, cut in half
3 apricots, pitted and diced
¼ cup chopped almonds
2 tablespoons freshly minced
parsley or mint
Salt and pepper to taste
Olive oil

cooking instructions

Place a coffee filter into a fine mesh sieve. Place the quinoa in the filter and rinse the quinoa under cold running water.

Heat the oil in a saucepan over medium heat. Add the quinoa and sauté for a few minutes, until it is slightly browned. Add the onion, mushrooms, ginger, and jalapeño, and sauté for 1 to 2 minutes. Add the turmeric, coriander, and cinnamon, and season with salt and pepper. Add 2 cups of water and bring to a boil. Reduce heat and simmer for 20 minutes or until the liquid is completely absorbed. Transfer the quinoa to a bowl and drizzle a little olive oil and squeeze some lemon juice over. Add the apricots, almonds, and parsley. Adjust seasoning and serve immediately.

Risotto with Olives

serves 8

ingredients

3 large tomatoes (about 1 pound)
1 tablespoon olive oil
1 small onion, diced
(about 4 ounces)
1 tablespoon minced garlic
12 ounces Arborio rice
4 ounces Chardonnay
1 teaspoon minced dried thyme
3 saffron threads

4 cups chicken stock
(low-fat and low-sodium)
¼ cup green olives, pitted
¼ cup grated Parmesan cheese
⅛ cup cream, heated
3 tablespoons minced fresh salad
herbs
Salt and pepper to taste

cooking instructions

Make a small X incision on the top and bottom of the tomatoes. Blanch the tomatoes for 20 seconds. Place in ice-cold water to stop the cooking process. Peel, seed, and dice the tomatoes.

Heat the oil in a pan over high heat. Add the onions and sauté until translucent. Add the garlic and rice, and stir for 1 minute. Add the wine, thyme, and saffron, then cook until the liquid is evaporated over medium heat. Add 2 cups of the stock and simmer uncovered. Once the liquid is absorbed, add the remaining 2 cups stock and the olives, and continue to simmer uncovered. Once the stock is almost absorbed, add the tomatoes, Parmesan cheese, cream, and salad herbs, then season to taste. Remove from heat and cover for 2 minutes before serving.

Salmon and Vegetable Carpaccio

serves 2

ingredients

6 ounces thinly sliced wild
smoked salmon
1 medium cucumber, peeled
(about 8 ounces)
1 large yellow squash, peeled
(about 8 ounces)

2 green onions, minced
2 teaspoons fresh dill, minced
4 tablespoons olive oil
1 lemon
Salt and pepper to taste

cooking instructions

Remove a couple of zest strips from the lemon and mince. Juice the lemon and set aside in a bowl. Add the olive oil, 1 teaspoon dill, half of the prepared zest, and season to taste.

Thinly slice the cucumber and yellow squash. Refrigerate until use. Equally divide the salmon in two plates, season to taste, and sprinkle with dill. Pour half the dressing over and refrigerate for 20 minutes. In the center of the salmon slices and in a round formation, alternate the cucumber and squash slices. Season lightly and garnish with the green onions, remaining zest and dill. Pour over the remaining dressing and serve immediately.

Sugar Snap Peas and Tuna Salad

serves 4

ingredients

For the salad:
4 ounces mesclun
1½ can of tuna in water, strained
(9 ounces)
1 large carrot, thinly sliced
(about 4 ounces)
2 large tomatoes, seeded and
diced
1 cup fresh sugar snap peas
(about 4 ounces)
Salt and pepper to taste

For the dressing:
1 shallot, minced
1 garlic clove, minced
3 tablespoons lemon juice
3 tablespoons olive oil
2 tablespoons salad herbs
Salt and pepper to taste

cooking instructions

Heat a steamer and add the sugar snap peas. Cook for 2 minutes. Add
the carrots and continue to steam for 2 minutes or until desired doneness.
In a bowl, mix the shallot, garlic, lemon juice, oil, and 1 tablespoon of
herbs, then season to taste. In a large bowl mix the mesclun with half of
the dressing. Add the tuna, tomatoes, carrot slices, and sugar snap peas.
Sprinkle with the remaining herbs and dressing before serving.

Fish & Seafood Entrées

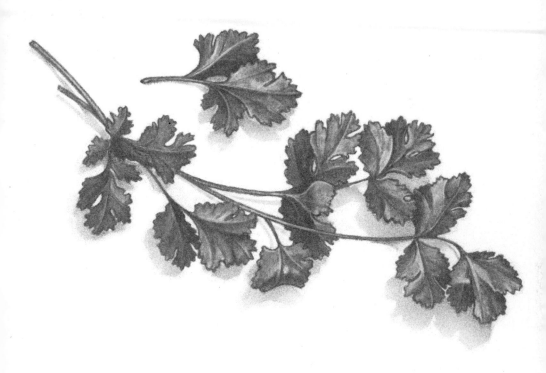

Steamed Salmon with Fennel

serves 4

ingredients

1 large salmon fillet (20 ounces)
1 medium onion, sliced
(about 6 ounces)
1 large carrot, sliced
(about 4 ounces)
1 teaspoon herbs de Provence
¼ cup vegetable stock
(low-fat and low-sodium)
1 teaspoon fennel seeds
Salt and pepper to taste

For the vegetables:
1 tablespoon olive oil
2 large fennel bulbs, trimmed and
sliced (about 1½ pounds)
1 medium onion, sliced
(about 6 ounces)
1 tablespoon garlic cloves,
minced
¼ cup vegetable stock
(low-fat and low-sodium)
Pinch cayenne pepper
Salt and pepper to taste

cooking instructions

Preheat the oven to 400°F.

For the fish: Prepare a large aluminum foil. Place the salmon in the middle. Sprinkle over a little salt, some pepper, and the herbs de Provence. Top with the onion, carrot, and a few fennel slices (see vegetables). Fold the aluminum foil a bit; add the stock, and fennel seeds. Close and place on a baking dish. Bake for 25 to 30 minutes, or until the salmon flesh starts to flake.

For the vegetables: Heat the oil in a nonstick pan over high heat. Add the onion and sauté until translucent. Add the fennel slices, garlic, and sauté for 2 minutes. Pour in the vegetable stock, cover, and cook for 15 to 20 minutes over low heat. Add the cayenne pepper and season to taste.

Place the salmon in a serving platter with its vegetables and juices, and serve immediately with the fennel.

Salmon with Orange Sauce

serves 4

ingredients

For the fish:
2 oranges
1 teaspoon canola oil
Four 5-ounce salmon fillets
1 teaspoon coriander seeds, crushed
1 shallot, thinly sliced
1½ cup fresh orange juice

1 tablespoon honey
1 tablespoon cornstarch, mixed with a little water
1 teaspoon dried parsley
Salt and pepper to taste

For the vegetables:
2 pounds asparagus, trimmed (about 32 asparagus spears)
½ orange, juiced
Salt and pepper to taste

cooking instructions

Preheat the oven to 400°F.

For the fish: Zest the two oranges and julienne the zest. Blanch them for 2 minutes. Remove and set aside. Remove the white pith from the oranges and slice the oranges (into approximately ⅜-inch slices).

Grease the bottom of a baking pan with the oil. Add the salmon and season lightly with pepper. Cover the fillets with a pinch of crushed coriander, half of the zest, the shallot, and the oranges slices. Warm up ¼ cup of the juice with the remaining coriander. Pour the juice mixture over the fish, cover the baking pan with aluminum foil, and bake for 20 minutes or until the flesh start to flake. Transfer the fish and solids to a serving platter. Cover with aluminum foil to keep warm. Pour the remaining liquid from the baking pan into a saucepan. Add the remaining zest and juice and the honey. Bring to a boil and reduce to ¾ cup. Thicken with cornstarch mixture, a little at a time, until the desired consistency is obtained. Strain and return the liquid to the pan, discarding solids. Add the parsley and season with salt. Pour the sauce over the fish.

For the vegetables: Prepare a steamer. Add the asparagus and cook for 2 to 3 minutes or to desired taste. Transfer the asparagus to a serving plate, sprinkle a little orange juice, and season to taste.

Broiled Salmon with Dill

serves 4

ingredients

Four 5-ounce salmon fillets
1 tablespoon olive oil
4 to 5 fresh dill branches, minced
Salt and pepper to taste

cooking instructions

Preheat the broiler. Rub olive oil over the flesh side of the fillets. Lightly season the fillets and spread the minced dill over them. Place the fillets on a greased pan, skin side up. Brush olive oil over the skin and broil for 3 to 4 minutes. Turn over and continue to broil for a few minutes or until the salmon flesh start to flake.

Spaghetti with Sun-Dried Tomatoes and Anchovies

serves 4

ingredients

12 ounces whole grain spaghetti
1 tablespoon olive oil
1 small onion, finely diced
(about 4 ounces)
1 tablespoon minced garlic
1 large green bell pepper, seeded,
ribs removed and diced medium
(about 6 ounces)
1 cup sun-dried tomatoes,
julienned

1 tablespoon capers, drained
2 ounces pitted Kalamata olives
1 teaspoon dried red pepper flakes
2 ounces canned anchovy fillets,
chopped, plus some oil
¼ cup fresh basil, chopped
3 tablespoons chopped fresh
parsley
2 tablespoons Parmesan cheese
Salt and pepper to taste

cooking instructions

Preheat the oven to 425°F.

Cook the spaghetti according to package directions. Strain, add a little bit of the oil from the anchovy can, mix, and set aside.

Heat the oil in a large nonstick pan over high heat. Add the onion and sauté until translucent. Add the garlic and bell pepper, then continue to cook for 3 minutes over medium heat. Add the sun-dried tomatoes, capers, olives, dried red pepper flakes, and anchovies. Sprinkle with pepper and continue to cook for 2 to 3 minutes. Mix in the pasta, herbs, and Parmesan cheese. Adjust seasoning and serve immediately.

Spicy Tuna with Avocado Spread

serves 4

ingredients

1 avocado, pureed
½ lime, juiced
4 tablespoons low-fat Greek yogurt
1 large jalapeño, seeded and diced
2 tablespoons cilantro
Four 5-ounce tuna fillets
1 tablespoon olive oil
1 large red onion, diced (about 8 ounces)

2 medium yellow bell peppers, seeded, ribs removed, and diced (about 12 ounces)
2 large Roma tomatoes, peeled and diced (about 12 ounces)
Salt to taste
Tabasco® sauce to taste
Cajun spices to taste

> ✔ *To peel the tomatoes: Make a small X incision on the top and bottom of the tomatoes. Blanch the tomatoes for 20 seconds. Place in ice-cold water to stop the cooking process. The tomatoes are now ready to peel.*

cooking instructions

Mix the avocado with the lime juice. Mix in the yogurt, jalapeno, and cilantro, and season with salt. Add Tabasco® and refrigerate until needed.

Preheat the broiler. Sprinkle Cajun spices on both sides of the fillets. Place the fillets on a baking sheet brushed with a little of the olive oil and broil for 2 to 3 minutes. Turnover and continue to broil 3 to 4 more minutes or until the fish flesh starts to flake. Adjust seasoning before serving.

Meanwhile, heat the remaining oil in a large pan over medium heat. Add the onion and sauté until translucent. Add the bell peppers and continue to sauté for 2 minutes. Mix in the tomatoes and cook for another 2 minutes. Add a little of the Cajun spices and salt.

Place the vegetables on a plate, top with the tuna and avocado spread, and serve immediately.

Broiled Tuna with Tarragon Sauce

serves 4

✔ *The cream can be substituted with Greek low-fat yogurt. If wine is not desired, substitute with stock. Serve with brown rice.*

ingredients

1 tablespoon olive oil
1 small shallot, minced
1 garlic clove, minced
½ cup white wine
(Sauvignon Blanc)
¾ cup vegetable stock
(low-fat and low-sodium)
8 fresh tarragon branches,
(4 branches minced, 4 whole)

2 tablespoons Dijon mustard
1 tablespoon cornstarch, mixed
with a little water
Four 5-ounce tuna fillets
Oil spray
2 tablespoons cream (optional)
Salt and pepper to taste

cooking instructions

Preheat the broiler. Heat the oil in a pan over high heat. Add the shallot and garlic, and sauté for 1 minute. Add the wine, stock, and half of the minced tarragon, and boil for 3 minutes. Strain and return liquid to the pan, discarding solids. Add the mustard and mix briefly. Add the cornstarch mixture, a little at a time, until the desired consistency is obtained. Remove from heat and set aside.

Place the fillets on a greased cookie sheet. Rub the whole tarragon branches on both sides of the fillets. Spray a little oil over the fillets and lightly season with pepper.

Broil for 4 to 5 minutes. Turn over and spray with a little more oil. Continue to broil until the flesh starts to flake. Remove the fillets and keep warm on a plate covered with aluminum foil. Reheat the prepared sauce, add the cream, if using, and the remaining minced tarragon, and bring to a boil. Season with salt and pepper and pour over the fillets. Serve immediately.

Tuna Spanish Style

serves 4

ingredients

Four 5-ounce tuna fillets
1 tablespoon olive oil
2 large onions, sliced
(about 1 pound)
6 large tomatoes
(about 2 pounds)
1 large green bell pepper; ribs
and seeds removed, sliced
(about 8 ounces)

1 tablespoon wheat flour
3 garlic cloves, minced
1 pinch dry thyme
1 pinch dry oregano
2 tablespoons fresh parsley,
minced
½ cup brown rice
Salt and pepper to taste

cooking instructions

Cook the rice according to package instructions. Make a small X incision on the top and bottom of the tomatoes. Blanch the tomatoes for 20 seconds. Place in ice-cold water to stop the cooking process. Peel, seed, and dice the tomatoes.

Heat 2 teaspoons of olive oil in a deep nonstick pan over high heat. Add the onions and sauté until translucent. Add the garlic, bell pepper, thyme, oregano, and sauté for 3 minutes over medium heat. Sprinkle with the flour and mix well. Add the tomatoes and continue to cook for 3 to 4 minutes.

Meanwhile, heat the remaining oil in a nonstick skillet over high heat. Add the fish and brown on both sides. Slide the fish into the vegetables, cover, and continue to cook for 15 to 20 minutes over low heat.

Transfer the fish to a serving platter. If necessary, thicken the sauce over medium heat. Add to the fish and serve immediately with the rice.

Grilled Sea Bass with Mango Salsa

serves 4

✔ *You can also broil the fillets for about the same amount of time.*

ingredients

2 mangos, diced
1 tomato, diced
1 small red onion, diced
2 green jalapenos, diced
1 bunch fresh cilantro, chopped
¼ cup lime juice

1½ tablespoons canola oil
Four 5-ounce sea bass fillets
Salt and pepper to taste

cooking instructions

In a bowl, mix the mangos, tomato, onion, jalapenos, cilantro, and lime juice. Season with salt and pepper and refrigerate at least 30 minutes.

Preheat a grill. Brush the oil over the fillets and season lightly with pepper. Grill the fish for 3 to 4 minutes skin side up. Turn over and continue to cook 3 to 4 minutes more or until the flesh starts to flake. Sprinkle a little salt and serve immediately with the mango salsa.

Sea Bass with Ginger and Lime

serves 4

ingredients

For the fish:
1 tablespoon olive oil
Four 5-ounce sea bass fillets
½ cup lime juice
½ small onion, diced
(about 2 ounces)
1 teaspoon minced garlic
1 tablespoon minced fresh ginger
½ cup Chardonnay wine (or other wine with lemon-lime tones)
1 tablespoon honey

1 teaspoon fresh rosemary
Cornstarch mixed with
a little water
2 tablespoons minced fresh parsley
Salt and pepper to taste

For the vegetables:
2 pounds chard, kale, spinach, beet greens, or mustard greens, cleaned and patted dry
1 lime, juiced
Salt and pepper to taste

cooking instructions

For the vegetables: Preheat a steamer. Add the greens and cook to desired tenderness. Remove greens and press out excess water. Chop, mix in some lime juice, and season with salt and pepper. Set aside.

For the fish: Heat the oil in a nonstick pan over medium heat. Lightly season the fillets with salt and pepper, add to the pan, and brown for two to three minutes. Turn over and cook for 2 minutes more. Add about ⅓ of the lime juice, cover, and reduce heat. Cook the fillets until the flesh starts to flake. Remove the fish from the pan and place on a serving platter. Cover with aluminum foil to keep warm. Add the onions, garlic, ginger, wine, remaining lime juice, honey, and rosemary to the pan. Mix well and bring to a boil. Reduce the sauce to ⅔ cup. Add a little of the cornstarch mixture and bring to a boil to thicken. Strain, discarding solids, and return to pan. Add the parsley and adjust seasoning. Pour over the fillets and serve immediately with the cooked greens.

Swordfish with Walnuts

serves 4

✔ *This walnut paste can be used as a dip for vegetables, for bruschetta, as a sandwich spread, salad dressing base, and much more.*

ingredients

For the fish:
1 slice wheat bread
4 tablespoons milk
½ cup walnuts
2 teaspoons minced garlic
1½ tablespoons olive oil
Pinch nutmeg
2 teaspoons canola oil
Four 5-ounce swordfish steaks
½ lemon, juiced
Salt and pepper to taste

For the vegetables:
3 large yellow squash, chopped (about 1 pound)
3 large tomatoes, quartered and seeded (about 1 pound)
1 teaspoon olive oil
1 teaspoon minced garlic
½ lemon, juiced
2 pinches dried Italian herbs
Salt and pepper to taste

cooking instructions

Preheat the oven to 425°F.

For the vegetables: In a casserole, toss the squash, tomatoes, oil, garlic, juice, and Italian herbs, and season with salt and pepper. Bake for 20 to 25 minutes, mixing halfway through the cooking time.

For the fish: Soak the bread in 1½ tablespoons of the milk. In a blender, puree the walnuts, garlic, olive oil, and nutmeg. Add the bread and mix well. Blend in 1½ tablespoons of the remaining milk and season with salt and pepper. Heat the oil in a nonstick pan over high heat. Lightly season the fish with pepper, add to the pan, and brown for two to three minutes. Turn over and sauté 2 minutes more. Add the juice, cover, reduce heat, and continue to cook for another 3 to 4 minutes or until the flesh start to flake. Sprinkle lightly with salt. Warm up the remaining 1 tablespoon milk and mix into the walnut paste. Serve immediately with the fish and vegetables.

Spanish-Style Sardines

serves 4

ingredients

For the fish:
8 whole sardines (about 2½ ounces)
2 tablespoons olive oil
1 small onion, finely diced
(about 4 ounces)
1 leek (white part only), diced small
1 small carrot, finely diced
(about 2 ounces)
1 large celery stalk, finely diced
(about 2 ounces)
1 tablespoon minced garlic
1 cup white wine (lemony Chardonnay
or Sauvignon Blanc)
1 lemon, zested and juiced

4 tablespoons sherry vinegar
1 bouquet garni
2 pinches paprika
½ cup vegetable stock
(low-sodium)
Salt and pepper to taste

For the vegetables:
1 tablespoon olive oil
1 pound pearl onions, peeled
1 teaspoon minced garlic
1 cup frozen baby lima beans
1 pinch Italian herbs
¼ cup vegetable stock
(low-sodium)
1 lemon, quartered
Salt and pepper to taste

cooking instructions

For the sardines: Remove the head and bones from the sardines (this can be done at the fish market). Heat 1 tablespoon of oil in a pan over high heat. Add the onions and leek, then cook for 2 minutes. Add the carrots, celery, garlic, wine, lemon zest and juice, vinegar, bouquet garni, and paprika, then cook for 10 minutes over medium heat. Add the stock and reduce by half. Season with salt and pepper and remove the bouquet garni.

Meanwhile, heat the remaining 1 tablespoon oil in a nonstick pan over medium heat. Lightly season the sardines with salt and pepper, add to the pan, and cook for 3 minutes or until cooked through. Do not turn over since they are small and very fragile. Transfer the sardines over a serving platter and spread the vegetables over.

For the vegetables: Heat the oil in a sauté pan over medium heat. Cook the pearl onions until golden brown. Add the garlic, lima beans, and Italian herbs, and season with salt and pepper. Add the stock, mix well, and bring to a boil. Continue to cook until the stock is almost evaporated. Adjust seasonings and transfer to a serving bowl. Serve with the prepared sardines and lemon wedges.

Stuffed Herring with Potato and Onion

serves 4

ingredients

4 small red potatoes
(about 3 ounces each)
1 teaspoon canola oil
1 large onion, sliced
(about 8 ounces)
1 tablespoon minced garlic
Four 4-ounce whole herring

2 teaspoons olive oil
1 bunch fresh parsley, minced
Dash white vinegar
Salt and pepper to taste

cooking instructions

Place the potatoes into a pan and cover with water. Add 1 teaspoon salt and bring to a boil over high heat. Reduce heat and simmer for 15 minutes. When just barely cooked, drain, and let cool. Peel and slice the potatoes.

Preheat the oven to 400°F.

Heat the canola oil in a nonstick pan over high heat. Add the onion and brown slightly. Add the garlic and continue to cook for 1 minute. Remove from heat and allow to cool.

Place each herring on its own piece of aluminum foil. Open the herring and sprinkle the cavities with a little pepper. Divide the potatoes and onions equally among the herring, place in the cavity and then close the herring. Sprinkle each herring with ½ teaspoon each of the olive oil and with a quarter of the parsley. Close the foils tight and place in a baking dish. Bake for 25 to 30 minutes. Serve immediately with a dash of white vinegar.

Mackerel with Garlic Cloves

serves 4

ingredients

For the fish:
Four 5-ounce whole mackerel
16 garlic cloves, peeled
2 tablespoons olive oil
Salt and pepper to taste

For the vegetables:
4 large carrots, sliced
(about 1 pound)
3 large zucchini, sliced
(about 1 pound)
1 lemon, quartered
Salt and pepper to taste

cooking instructions

Preheat the oven to 400°F.

For the fish: Sprinkle a little salt and some pepper inside the mackerel cavities. Grease the bottom of a baking pan with a little of the oil. Blanch the garlic cloves in boiling water for 3 minutes. Slightly crush them on the bottom of the greased pan. Top them with the mackerel and drizzle the remaining oil over the fish. Bake for 20 to 25 minutes.

For the vegetables: Preheat a steamer. Add the carrots and cook for 4 minutes. Add the zucchini and continue to cook for 2 to 3 minutes or to desired doneness. Transfer to a serving platter and season to taste.

Serve the mackerel with the vegetables and lemon wedges.

Greek-Style Cod Fish

serves 4

ingredients

3 large tomatoes (about 1 pound)
Four 5-ounce cod fillets
2 tablespoons olive oil
1 large onion, diced
(about 8 ounces)
2 medium zucchini, diced
(about 8 ounces)
1 medium eggplant, peeled and
diced (about 8 ounces)
1 large red bell pepper, seeded,
ribs removed, and diced
(about 6 ounces)

1 large yellow bell pepper, seeded,
ribs removed, and diced (about
6 ounces)
1 tablespoon minced garlic
1 bay leaf
½ teaspoon Italian herbs
3 tablespoons minced fresh
parsley
5 fresh basil leaves, minced
4 ounces feta cheese, diced
Salt and pepper to taste

cooking instructions

Make a small X incision at the top of the tomatoes. Heat some water over high heat and bring to a boil. Blanch the tomatoes for 20 seconds. Remove and place in ice-cold water to stop the cooking process. Peel, seed, and dice the tomatoes.

Heat 1 tablespoon of the oil in a deep pan over medium heat. Add the onion and sauté until translucent. Add the zucchini, eggplant, bell peppers, garlic, tomatoes, bay leaf, and Italian herbs, then bring to a boil. Reduce heat, cover, and cook for 20 minutes.

Heat the remaining 1 tablespoon oil in a nonstick skillet over medium heat. Lightly season the fillets with salt and pepper, add to the pan and brown for two to three minutes. Turn over and sauté for two minutes more. Slide the fillets into the vegetables and continue to cook uncovered for 15 minutes. Remove the fish from the pan and place on a serving platter. Cover with aluminum foil to keep warm. If the vegetable stew is thin, reduce a little more, uncovered, over medium heat. Add the parsley and basil, then season to taste. Transfer to a serving bowl, add the feta cheese, and serve immediately with the fillets.

Shrimp Scampi Style

serves 4

ingredients

4 tablespoons olive oil

2 pounds large shrimp, shelled and de-veined

2 medium red bell peppers; seeded, ribs removed, and sliced (about 12 ounces)

4 large garlic cloves, minced

½ lemon with its zest set aside

2 tablespoons freshly minced basil

½ cup whole wheat pasta

Salt and pepper to taste

cooking instructions

Cook the pasta according to package directions. Heat the oil and garlic in a large pan over medium heat. Add the shrimp and cook for 1 minute or until fully cooked, stirring occasionally. Add the bell peppers, lemon juice, lemon peel, basil, and season to taste. Continue to cook for 2 minutes or until the shrimp are cooked through, stirring occasionally. Add the cooked pasta and serve immediately.

Scallops with Tangerines

serves 4

ingredients

1 tablespoon olive oil

1 pound scallops

6 tangerines

1 cup orange juice

1 teaspoon minced ginger

1 shallot, minced

8 ounces mushrooms

2 tablespoons parsley, minced

Olive oil

Salt and pepper to taste

cooking instructions

Peel and segment the tangerines. Place the orange juice and half of the ginger in a saucepan and bring to a boil over high heat. Reduce until you end up with ¼ cup and set aside.

Heat 1 teaspoon of olive oil in a saucepan over high heat. Add the mushrooms, shallot, remaining ginger, and sauté quickly. Add parsley and season to taste.

Meanwhile, lightly season the scallops. Heat 2 teaspoons of olive oil in a large saucepan over high heat. Add the scallops and sear on both sides. Add the mandarin segments, reduced orange juice, and continue to sauté for 1 minute. Serve immediately with the mushrooms and drizzle with a little olive oil.

Meat, Poultry & Vegetable Entrées

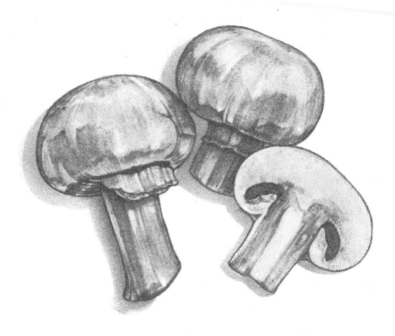

Chicken Cacciatore

serves 6

ingredients

2 tablespoons olive oil

One 4-pound roasting chicken, cut into serving pieces

¼ cup chicken stock (low-fat and low-sodium)

1 medium onion, diced (about 6 ounces)

1 large carrot, diced (about 4 ounces)

2 celery stalks, diced (about 4 ounces)

1 medium green bell pepper, diced (about 6 ounces)

2 garlic cloves, minced

1 cup canned diced tomatoes

1 cup mushrooms, sliced

Couple pinches of dry Italian herbs

½ cup wild rice

Salt and pepper to taste

cooking instructions

Preheat the oven to 300°F. Heat a third of the oil in a large pan over high heat. Add half the chicken pieces and brown on all sides. Transfer to a large deep ovenproof pan and repeat the process with a third of the oil and remaining chicken pieces. Deglaze the pan with a little chicken stock and, with a whisk scrape all of the particles from the bottom and sides of the pan. Add liquid and particles to the chicken. Add remaining oil and slightly brown the onion. Add the carrot, celery, garlic, tomatoes, mushrooms, herbs, and bring to a boil over medium heat. Season to taste and transfer to the chicken pan. Cover with aluminum foil and bake for 40 to 45 minutes.

Meanwhile, cook the wild rice according to package directions. Serve with the prepared chicken when done.

Lemon Chicken

serves 4

> ✔ *This lemon chicken can also be used for appetizers, salads, soups, etc...*

ingredients

3 tablespoons olive oil
Four 4-ounce skinless chicken breasts
5 lemons
1 tablespoon fresh poultry herbs
Salt and pepper to taste

cooking instructions

Juice four lemons. Mix in two tablespoons of olive oil, the herbs, and season with pepper. Place the chicken pieces in a plastic bag. Pour the lemon marinade over the chicken and refrigerate for at least one hour, rotating every 10 minutes.

Preheat the broiler. Remove the chicken breasts from the marinade and pat dry. Place them on a greased cookie sheet and brush a little olive oil over each breast. Broil for approximately 6 to 7 minutes on each side. Watch carefully to avoid burning. Serve immediately with lemon wedges.

Chicken Breast with Dijon Mustard

serves 4

ingredients

Four 5-ounce skinless chicken breasts
1 tablespoon Dijon mustard
2 teaspoons lemon juice
½ teaspoon garlic powder
Canola oil
Salt and pepper to taste

cooking instructions

Preheat the oven to 375 °F. Place the chicken breasts in a lightly oiled pan. In a bowl, mix the mustard, lemon juice, and garlic powder. Spread over the chicken breasts and season to taste. Bake for 20 to 25 minutes, or until cooked through. Time may vary depending on the thickness of the breasts.

Chicken Burgers
with Lettuce Wraps

serves 2

ingredients

Four 4-ounce chicken burgers
4 garlic cloves, minced
4 tablespoons low-calorie Caesar dressing
2 white anchovy fillets
16 lettuce leaves
4 tablespoons Parmesan Cheese Canola oil
Salt and pepper to taste

cooking instructions

In a food processor puree the anchovy fillet with the dressing. Add a little water to thin out. Lightly season the burgers and shape them to fit in the lettuce leaves. Do not allow the meat to touch the leaves. Heat 2 tablespoons of olive oil with the minced garlic. Remove once boiling and set aside. Preheat the grill on medium high heat. Don't forget to grease the grill before adding the burgers. Cook them for 3 to 5 minutes on each side or until cooked through.

Meanwhile, carefully brush the garlic oil over the lettuce leaves.

Place two leaves on a plate, top with one burger, spread 1 Tbsp. Caesar dressing, sprinkle with cheese and fold a bit over thetop. Top with 2 more leaves and tuck underneath to seal. Serve immediately with your favorite accompaniment. You may use toothpick to hold for presentation.

Garlic Chicken

serves 4

ingredients

2 pinches coarse salt
8 to 10 garlic cloves, minced
4 teaspoons olive oil
1 tablespoon dried Italian herbs
Four 6-ounces bone-in, skin-on chicken breasts
1 large lemon, cut in 8 slices
Pepper to taste

cooking instructions

Preheat the oven to 375°F. Sprinkle the coarse salt over the minced garlic cloves. Press the side of a chef's knife into the mixture until you end up with smooth paste. Transfer to a bowl. Mix in the olive oil, Italian herbs, and season with pepper. With your fingers, carefully separate the chicken skin slightly from the flesh, being careful not to break the skin. Spread the garlic mixture over the chicken flesh, add 2 lemon slices per breast, and push back the skin. Place the breasts in a baking dish and bake for 20 to 25 minutes, or until cooked through. Time may vary depending on the thickness of the breasts. Serve immediately and remember to discard the skin when eating.

Chicken Breast with Asian Glaze

serves 4

ingredients

Four 5-ounce chicken breasts
with bones and skin
2 tablespoons maple syrup
1 tablespoon green tea leaves
1 tablespoon Oriental
hot mustard

1 garlic clove, minced
2 tablespoons sesame seeds
1 teaspoon ground ginger
Canola oil
Salt and pepper to taste

cooking instructions

Preheat the oven to 350°F. Wash and pat dry the chicken breasts. Carefully pass your fingers between the meat and the skin to loosen up the skin without breaking it.

Heat the maple syrup, tea, mustard, garlic, and ginger in a saucepan over low heat until well blended. Season to taste and set aside. Lift up the chicken skin and brush the mixture over the chicken meat. Sprinkle the sesame seeds under the skin. Brush canola oil over the skin and roast for 30 minutes, or until cooked through. Remove skin before serving.

Cornish Hen with Red Cabbage

serves 4

ingredients

2 tablespoons grapeseed oil
2 Cornish hens
4 slices turkey bacon
1 large onion, sliced
(about 8 ounces)
2 Granny Smith apple, sliced
(about 8 ounces)
1 red cabbage, sliced
(about 1 ½ pounds)

4 cups chicken stock (low-fat and
low-sodium)
2 cloves
1 laurel leaf
1 teaspoon caraway seeds
Mustard
Salt and pepper to taste

cooking instructions

Blanch the red cabbage into boiling salted water. Rinse the Cornish hen
under cold water, pat dry, and lightly season.

Heat half of the oil in a sauté pan. Sear the Cornish hen on all sides
(about 10 minutes).

Heat the remaining oil in a Dutch oven or brasier. Add the bacon, onion,
apples, and sweat for two minutes. Add the red cabbage, stock, cloves,
laurel leaf, caraway seeds, and bring to boil. Top with the Cornish hen,
cover, and cook for 40 to 50 minutes in the oven. Serve with mustard on
the side.

Turkey Breast with Italian Herbs

serves 8

✔ *Great way to prepare your own turkey breast meat for salads, snacks, soups, etc… You can also vary the flavoring by using different herbs. Sage is great and soothing.*

ingredients

1 tablespoon olive oil
2 pounds turkey breast (with skin)
4 teaspoons Italian herbs
Bunch of fresh basil leaves
¼ cup chicken stock (low-fat and low-sodium)
Salt and pepper to taste

cooking instructions

Preheat the oven to 350° F. Mix 1 tablespoon of Italian herbs with a little pepper. Spread all over the turkey breast under its skin. Add as many basil leaves as you can fit under the skin without tearing the skin. Brush olive oil over the skin.

Place the turkey breast skin side up in a roasting pan. Pour ¼ cup of chicken stock in the pan, add the remaining Italian herbs, and bake for an hour or until a meat thermometer registers 180° F. Keep moistening with chicken stock. To keep the turkey breast moist, do not allow the pan to get dry. Transfer the turkey breast to a platter and let cool before slicing.

Turkey Meatloaf with Tomato Sauce

serves 6

> ✓ *Suggestion: Serve with steamed vegetables such as broccoli and yellow squash.*

ingredients

1 teaspoon olive oil
1 small onion, minced
(about 4 ounces)
1 celery stalk, minced
(about 2 ounces)
2 garlic cloves, minced
1 pound ground buffalo meat
¾ pound ground chicken or turkey meat
3 ounces ground oats
1 large egg, beaten

3 ounces chicken stock
(low-fat and low-sodium)
1 teaspoon salt
¼ teaspoon pepper
¼ teaspoon dry mustard
⅛ teaspoon dry sage
½ teaspoon dry Italian herbs
10 ounces diced tomato

For serving: Your favorite tomato sauce (about 1 cup)

cooking instructions

Preheat the oven to 350°F. Heat the oil in a pan over high heat. Add the onion, celery, garlic, and cook for 2 minutes. Transfer to a mixing bowl and add the remaining ingredients. Mix well and place the meatloaf into a greased loaf pan. Bake the loaf for 1 hour to 1½ hours or until cooked through. Serve with your favorite tomato sauce.

If buffalo meat is not available, substitute with organic sirloin groun d beef.

Turkey Chili

serves 4

ingredients

1 teaspoon canola oil
1 large onion, diced
(about 8 ounces)
1 medium green bell pepper;
cored, seeded, and diced
(about 6 ounces)
2 garlic cloves, minced
1 pound ground turkey
15 ounces canned diced tomatoes
2 ounces tomato paste

1¼ cups chicken stock
(low-fat and low-sodium)
12 ounces cooked kidney beans or
pinto beans
1 teaspoon dried thyme
1 teaspoon dried oregano
2 teaspoons ground cumin
2 tablespoons chili powder
¼ teaspoon cayenne pepper
Salt to taste

cooking instructions

Heat the oil in a deep pan over medium heat. Add the meat and
brown slightly. Remove the excess fat rendered by the meat. Add
the onion, pepper, and garlic, then mix well. Stir in the tomatoes,
tomato paste, stock, herbs, and spices. Bring to a boil and reduce
heat. Simmer uncovered for 30 to 40 minutes. Stir occasionally and
thicken longer, if necessary. Add the beans and bring to a simmer.
Adjust seasoning and serve immediately.

Venison with Spicy Raspberry Sauce

serves 4

ingredients

1 cup raspberries

4 teaspoons grapeseed oil

Four 4-ounce venison steaks

1 large shallot, minced

½ teaspoon black peppercorns, crushed

2 pinches dried thyme

4 tablespoons aged balsamic vinegar

1 cup Cabernet Sauvignon

4 tablespoons demi-glace (if not available, use brown sauce)

2 tablespoons freshly minced parsley

Salt and pepper to taste

cooking instructions

In a food processor, puree half the raspberries. Pass through a sieve and set aside.

Heat the oil in a nonstick pan over medium-high heat. Lightly season the venison steaks with pepper, add to the pan, and sauté until golden brown. Turn over and continue to cook 2 to 3 minutes more. Transfer the steaks to a plate and cover with aluminum foil to keep warm. Add the shallots, peppercorns, thyme, vinegar, wine, and raspberry sauce, and deglaze the pan. Bring to a boil and reduce liquid by half. Add demi-glace and steak juices, then season with salt and pepper. Bring to a boil, add the steaks, and the remaining whole raspberries, and continue to simmer for a minute. Serve immediately.

Lamb Chops with Garlic Spread

serves 4

ingredients

4 cups green beans
(about 2 pounds)
6 teaspoons olive oil
2 tablespoons minced garlic
2 teaspoons freshly minced
parsley

2 teaspoons freshly minced
rosemary
½ teaspoon dry crushed
red pepper
Four 4-ounce loin lamb chops
Salt and pepper to taste

cooking instructions

Trim and place the green beans in a pan. Cover with water, add 1
teaspoon of salt, and bring to boil. Reduce heat and simmer until tender.
Drain and transfer to a serving bowl. Add 2 teaspoons olive oil, season
with salt and pepper, and mix well.

In a bowl, mix 2 teaspoons of the remaining oil, the garlic, parsley,
rosemary, and dry crushed red pepper. Rub the spread over the lamb
chops.

Heat the remaining 2 teaspoons oil in a nonstick pan over medium heat.
Add the lamb chops and cook for 3 to 4 minutes on each side or to
desired doneness. Serve immediately with the prepared green beans.

Duck Breast with Berries

serves 6

✓ *25% or more of fat will be discarded during the cooking process. The amount of fat may vary depending on the type of breast you get.*

ingredients

½ cup wild rice
Four 6-ounce duck breasts
1 teaspoon grapeseed oil
1 shallot, sliced
2 tablespoons red wine vinegar
½ cup Zinfandel or Syrah
1 cup chicken stock (low-fat and low-sodium)

8 ounces blueberries
1 fresh thyme branch
1 fresh rosemary sprig
2 juniper berries
Cornstarch mixed with a little water
Salt and pepper to taste

cooking instructions

Cook the rice according to package instructions. Heat the oil in an ovenproof sauté pan over high heat. Lightly season the underside of the duck breasts with salt and pepper, add to the pan skin side down, and sauté until golden brown, approximately 3 minutes. Turn over and cook for 2 minutes more. Place in the oven for 5 minutes (rare) to 10 minutes (well-done). Remove the breasts from the pan and place on a serving platter. Cover with aluminum foil to keep warm.

Discard excess fat from the pan. Add the shallot, vinegar, and wine, and boil until reduced by half. Add the stock, half of the blueberries, the thyme, rosemary, and juniper berries, and boil until reduced by half. Pass through a sieve, pressing hard to extract all the juices, and return the liquid to the pan. Add any juices rendered by the duck breasts and bring to a boil. Reduce a little more and thicken with a little cornstarch mixture. Adjust seasonings and add the remaining blueberries. Bring to a boil and pour over the duck breasts. Serve immediately with the wild rice.

Tofu and Collard Greens Burgers

serves 4

ingredients

8 ounces tofu
6 ounces cooked collard greens
1 small onion, diced
(about 4 ounces)
1 small carrot, shredded
(about 2 ounces)
2 scallions, chopped
2 garlic cloves, minced
1⅓ cups water crackers

4 teaspoons almond butter
2 tablespoons minced salad herbs
4 slices of cheddar cheese
(about 4 ounces)
Salt and pepper to taste

cooking instructions

Mix all the ingredients, except cheese, in a food processor until well combined. Form 4 patties and grill on each side for 4 to 5 minutes. Melt the cheese on top and serve immediately.

Mediterranean Portobello Burger

serves 4

ingredients

4 teaspoons olive oil

4 large portobello mushrooms caps

4 slices onion

2 garlic cloves, minced

4 tablespoons roasted red bell pepper spread

4 teaspoons chopped black olives

4 teaspoons feta cheese

8 slices tomato

8 large basil leaves

Lettuce leaves wide enough to wrap portobello mushrooms

Apple cider vinegar

Pepper to taste

cooking instructions

Preheat the grill to medium heat.

Brush 1 teaspoon olive oil and sprinkle pepper over each portobello. Grill the mushrooms for 2 minutes on each side. Add the onion and grill. Turn the mushrooms so that the top of the mushroom cap is on the grill. Fill the underside cavity with the garlic, bell pepper spread, and olives, and season with salt and pepper. Grill for another minute or two.

Place each portobello mushroom on a few lettuce leaves (cap side down), add 1 teaspoon feta cheese, 1 grilled onion slice, 2 slices tomato, 2 basil leaves, and sprinkle vinegar. Close the lettuce leaves to seal and serve immediately.

Tofu with Stir-Fried Vegetables

serves 4

ingredients

2 teaspoons canola oil
1 medium onion, sliced
(about 6 ounces)
2 medium carrots, thinly sliced on
the diagonal (about 6 ounces)
3 large garlic cloves, minced
1 inch ginger, minced
Florets from 1 large head broccoli
(about 8 ounces)
1 medium red bell pepper, seeded,
ribs removed, and sliced
(about 6 ounces)
4 baby bok choy, sliced
½ cup sugar snap peas
(about 2½ ounces)

2 teaspoons Chinese five-spice
powder
12 ounces firm tofu, diced
1 cup soy sprouts (about 3 ounces)
2 tablespoons freshly minced
parsley
2 tablespoons freshly minced
cilantro
¼ cup soy sauce mixed with
2 teaspoons cornstarch
1 teaspoon sesame oil
1 tablespoon sesame seeds
Pepper to taste

cooking instructions

Heat the oil in a large wok or saucepan over high heat. Add the onion
and cook until translucent. Add the carrots, garlic, and ginger, and cook
until the carrots are tender. Add the broccoli, bell pepper, bok choy,
sugar snap peas, and five-spice powder, and cook for 2 minutes. Add the
tofu, sprouts, parsley, and cilantro, and cook for 1 minute. Mix the soy
sauce and cornstarch together. Add the mixture to the prepared food
and mix well while thickening. Add the sesame oil and sesame seeds.
Season with pepper and serve immediately.

Side Dishes & Snacks

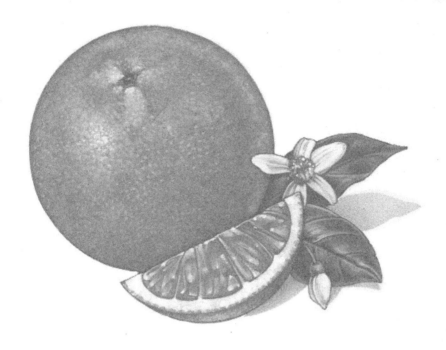

Stuffed Eggplant

serves 4

ingredients

1 egg
½ cup wheat breadcrumbs
½ teaspoon dried Italian herbs,
minced
2 medium eggplants
(about 1 pound)
Olive oil

1 medium onion, diced
(about 6 ounces)
2 tablespoons minced garlic
4 basil leaves, minced
¼ cup minced fresh parsley
Salt and pepper to taste

cooking instructions

Place the egg in a saucepan and cover with water. Bring to a boil over medium heat and cook for 10 minutes. Drain and cool in cold water. Peel the egg and mash with a fork in a bowl. Meanwhile, mix the breadcrumbs and dried Italian herbs.

Preheat the oven to 425°F. Cut the eggplants in half and remove the flesh without damaging the skin. Make very small incisions on the rim tops to allow the skin to stretch a bit, this will prevent breakage during cooking. Place the eggplant halves in a small greased baking pan and brush them with oil. Set aside. In a food processor puree the eggplant flesh and mashed egg. Heat 1 teaspoon oil in a nonstick pan over medium heat. Add the onions and garlic, then sauté for 2 minutes. Add the eggplant mixture and fresh herbs, then cook for 2 minutes more. Season with salt and pepper and fill the eggplant cavities with this mixture. Sprinkle the herbed breadcrumbs over the eggplant halves and sprinkle with a little olive oil. Bake for 30 to 35 minutes.

Marinated Vegetables with Lemon

serves 4

ingredients

For marinade:
1 lemon, zest removed and juiced
1 tablespoon minced garlic
1 branch fresh thyme, minced
1 teaspoon honey
1 tablespoon rice vinegar
3 tablespoons olive oil
1 teaspoon dried parsley
Salt and pepper to taste

For the vegetables:
2 large carrots (about 8 ounces)
1 large onion (about 8 ounces)
8 asparagus spears
(about 8 ounces)
Florets from 1 medium head
broccoli (about 8 ounces)

cooking instructions

For the marinade: In a bowl, mix all the marinade ingredients together and set aside.

For the vegetables: Cut the vegetables the same size for even cooking. Parboil the carrots for 2 minutes and place immediately in ice-cold water to stop the cooking process.

Place all the vegetables in a plastic bag, add the marinade, mix well, and refrigerate for a minimum of 4 hours.

Preheat the oven to 450°F. Transfer the vegetables and marinade to a baking pan. Bake for 20 to 25 minutes or to desired tenderness.

White Bean Stew

serves 8

ingredients

2 pounds dried white beans
1 teaspoon olive oil
1 medium onion, diced
(about 6 ounces)
1 medium carrot, diced
(about 3 ounces)
2 medium celery stalks, diced
(about 3 ounces)
2 tablespoons minced garlic

1 tablespoon all-purpose baking
flour
1 bouquet garni
4 cups chicken stock (low-fat and
low-sodium)
One 15-ounce can tomato puree
2 tablespoons freshly minced
parsley
Salt and pepper to taste

cooking instructions

Place the beans in a large stockpot and add enough water to cover them. Bring to a boil over high heat. Remove from heat and let stand covered for 30 minutes. Drain the beans and rinse under cold water.

Heat the oil in a large pan over high heat. Add the onion, carrot, celery stalks, and garlic, then sauté for 2 minutes. Mix in the flour. Add the beans, bouquet garni, and 4 cups of stock. If the beans are not covered, add enough water to do so. Bring to a boil, reduce heat, and simmer covered for 1 to 1½ hours, or until tender. Add the tomato purée and bring to a boil. Add parsley and season to taste. If the mixture is too thin, remove some beans, mash them, and add them back to the stew. Serve immediately.

Eggplant Mediterranean Style

serves 4

✓ *If ground thyme and oregano are difficult to find, use fresh versions and mince as small as possible.*

ingredients

2 small eggplants, both ends trimmed (about 1 pound)
1 tablespoon paprika
1 tablespoon ground ginger
1 tablespoon garlic powder
1 teaspoon coriander
1 teaspoon cumin

½ teaspoon cayenne pepper
¼ teaspoon ground thyme
¼ teaspoon ground oregano
2 tablespoons olive oil
Salt to taste

cooking instructions

Cut eggplant slices lengthwise and arrange on baking sheet. Mix all the spices together. On both sides of the eggplant slices, brush olive oil, season with salt, and sprinkle the prepared spices. Preheat the broiler or barbecue. Broil or grill until golden brown, about 2 minutes per side.

Zucchini and Bell Peppers with Pine Nuts

serves 4

ingredients

1 tablespoon olive oil
1 small onion, sliced
(about 4 ounces)
2 zucchini, sliced
(about 12 ounces)
2 red bell peppers, sliced
(about 12 ounces)

2 pinches dried Italian herbs
¼ cup pine nuts
Salt and pepper to taste

cooking instructions

Heat the oil in a large pan over high heat. Add the onion and sauté until translucent. Add the zucchini, bell peppers, and herbs, and sauté over medium heat until slightly browned and cooked through. Mix occasionally to avoid burning. Add the pine nuts and season with salt and pepper.

Spinach with Walnuts and Pomegranate

serves 4

ingredients

6 tablespoons pomegranate juice
3 tablespoons plus 3 teaspoons olive oil
6 cups fresh spinach
¼ cup walnuts, chopped
4 tablespoons pomegranate seeds
Pinch of nutmeg
Salt and pepper to taste

cooking instructions

Place the pomegranate juice in a pan and bring to boil. Reduce to 2 tablespoons and let cool.

In a large bowl, mix the 3 tablespoons of oil, the reduced pomegranate juice, and the nutmeg. Season with salt and pepper and set aside.

Heat 1½ teaspoons of oil in a large skillet over medium heat. Add 3 cups of the spinach and sauté until barely wilted. Transfer the spinach to a platter. Heat the remaining 1½ teaspoons oil and add the remaining 3 cups of the spinach and sauté until barely wilted. Add the first batch back to the pan, then blend in the pomegranate vinaigrette. Transfer to a serving platter, sprinkle the walnuts and pomegranate seeds, and serve immediately.

Wild Smoked Salmon Roll

serves 1

ingredients

12 asparagus spears, trimmed
(about 12 ounces asparagus)
3 ounces smoked wild salmon
(about 4 slices)
4 tablespoons Shallot and Chives
Boursin® Cheese (regular)
Pepper to taste

✔ *This may be served with a small salad on the side for a light lunch meal.*

You can substitute the Boursin® cheese with a mild goat cheese. Add freshly minced chives and a little lemon juice to thin out.

cooking instructions

Preheat a steamer over high heat. Add the asparagus, reduce heat, and cook until desired tenderness. Remove from the steamer and blanch in ice-cold water to stop the cooking process.

Lay each smoked salmon slice on a large cutting board. Spread 1 tablespoon of Boursin® over each slice. Add 3 asparagus per slice, sprinkle with pepper to taste, and roll. Serve immediately or refrigerate until needed.

Vegetarian Chili

serves 4

ingredients

1 tablespoon canola oil or olive oil

2 medium onions, chopped (about 12 ounces)

2 garlic cloves, minced

1 large green bell pepper, seeded, ribs removed, and diced (about 8 ounces)

1 large red bell pepper, seeded, ribs removed, and diced (about 8 ounces)

1 large zucchini, diced (about 8 ounces)

1 large yellow squash, diced (about 8 ounces)

2 large portobello mushrooms, diced

One 15-ounce can diced tomatoes

1 ½ cups vegetable stock (low-fat and low-sodium)

2 tablespoons chili powder

2 teaspoons ground cumin

¼ teaspoon cayenne pepper

1 teaspoon dried thyme

1 teaspoon dried oregano

1 tablespoon cornstarch, mixed with a little water

12 ounces corn kernels (canned or cut from fresh corn)

3 cups cooked kidney beans or pinto beans (canned or home cooked)

Salt to taste

cooking instructions

Warm the oil in a deep pan over medium heat. Add the onions and garlic, then sauté for 2 minutes. Add the bell peppers, zucchini, yellow squash, mushrooms, tomatoes, stock, spices, and herbs, then bring to a boil. Reduce heat and simmer until the vegetables are tender, about 5 minutes. Pass through a sieve, set the vegetables aside, and return the liquids to the pan. Reduce over high heat to concentrate the flavors and season with salt and pepper. If needed, thicken with a little cornstarch water mixture. Return the vegetables to the reduced liquid, add corn and beans, bring to a boil, and serve immediately.

Swiss Chard Tagine

serves 4

ingredients

2 pounds Swiss chard
2 tablespoons olive oil
1 small onion, diced (about 4 ounces)
1 tablespoon garlic cloves, minced
Salt, pepper, and paprika to taste

cooking instructions

Wash the Swiss chard and blanch in simmering salted water for 2 minutes. Strain and press out excess water. Let cool and chop.

Heat the oil in a nonstick pan over high heat. Add the onion and garlic, then sauté for 2 minutes. Add the Swiss chard and cook for 5 minutes, or until tender. Sprinkle with salt, pepper, and paprika to taste. Mix well and serve immediately.

Provençal-Style Baked Tomatoes

serves 4

> ✔ *Because anchovy is very salty, there is no salt in this recipe.*

ingredients

¼ cup breadcrumbs
¼ teaspoon herbes de Provence (or Italian herbs)
4 large tomatoes
4 teaspoons anchovy paste
2 tablespoons olive oil
2 tablespoons minced garlic

4 large pinches freshly minced basil
¼ cup grated Parmesan
Pepper to taste

cooking instructions

Preheat the oven to 375°F.

Thoroughly mix the breadcrumbs with the herbs. Cut the tomatoes in half. On each half, spread a little anchovy paste and sprinkle ¼ teaspoon oil. Add garlic and pepper to taste. Sprinkle the basil, breadcrumbs mixture, and Parmesan.

Place in a baking dish and bake for 20 to 25 minutes. Serve immediately.

Cottage Cheese, Raisins, and Walnuts

> ✓ *Option: Sprinkle pomegrante seeds.*

serves 1

ingredients

⅓ cup low-fat cottage cheese, cold
1 tablespoon chopped walnuts
2 teaspoons raisins
Cinnamon to taste

cooking instructions

Mix cottage cheese, walnut, and raisins. Sprinkle with cinnamon to taste and serve immediately.

Green Beans with Mushrooms

serves 4

ingredients

1 pound green beans, ends trimmed
1½ tablespoons olive oil
1 small onion, sliced (about 4 ounces)
½ cup mushrooms, sliced
2 garlic cloves, minced

2 pinches minced fresh thyme
2 tablespoons minced fresh basil
1 tablespoon minced fresh parsley
Salt and pepper to taste

cooking instructions

Place the green beans in a large pan and fill with enough water to cover them. Add 1 teaspoon of salt and bring to a boil over high heat. Reduce heat and simmer until cooked through. Drain and set aside.

Heat 1 tablespoon of oil in a nonstick pan over medium heat. Add the onion and sauté until translucent. Add the garlic, mushrooms, and herbs, then sauté for 2 minutes. Blend in the green beans and remaining oil. Season with salt and pepper, and serve immediately.

Wild Rice with Vegetables

serves 8

ingredients

1⅓ cups wild rice

2 teaspoons olive oil

2 medium onions, finely diced
(about 12 ounces)

2 medium carrots, finely diced
(about 6 ounces)

3 large celery stalks, finely diced
(about 6 ounces)

1 garlic clove, minced

4 cups vegetables stock

2 tablespoons minced fresh
parsley

Salt and pepper to taste

cooking instructions

Rinse the rice well and drain. Heat the oil in a deep pan over high heat.
Add the onions, carrots, celery, and garlic, and sauté for 2 minutes. Add
the rice and sauté for 1 minute. Add the stock and parsley, and bring
to a boil. Cover, reduce heat, and cook until tender (approximately 45
minutes but it may depend of the type of rice you use. For best results,
see package instructions). Season with salt and pepper and remove from
heat. If necessary, strain and serve immediately.

Roasted Pumpkin

serves 4

✓ *You can also use the cooked pumpkin to make a purée or soup. Thin out with low-fat milk until the necessary consistency is reached. You can also use the cooked pumpkin as a base for dips or as a dessert base.*

ingredients

3 pounds sugar pumpkin
1 tablespoon grapeseed oil
Pumpkin pie spices mix
Salt and pepper to taste

cooking instructions

Cut open the pumpkin, remove seeds and clean the inside with a spoon. Brush oil inside the cavity, season to taste, and place opening side down on a baking sheet. Roast for 30 to 45 minutes or until tender. Cut out and sprinkle with a little pumpkin pie spices before serving.

Roasted Potatoes with Artichokes

serves 4

ingredients

8 ounces frozen baby artichokes
4 medium red potatoes, quartered
(about one pound)
2 medium onions, quartered
(about 12 ounces)
2 large tomatoes, quartered
(about 12 ounces)

2 garlic cloves, minced
1 tablespoon lemon juice
3 tablespoons olive oil
1 teaspoon freshly minced
rosemary
Salt and pepper to taste

cooking instructions

Preheat the oven to 425°F.

Cook the artichokes according to package directions and set aside.

Heat 2 tablespoons of olive oil in a pan over high heat. Add the garlic, rosemary, and lemon juice. Sauté briefly and remove from heat. Let stand for 5 minutes and strain. Place the potatoes and onions in a baking dish and mix in the flavored oil. Season to taste and bake for 35 minutes. Remove from the oven, add the artichokes, tomatoes, adjust seasoning, and continue to cook for 10 minutes. Drizzle with a little hot olive oil before serving.

Peaches with Part-Skim Ricotta

serves 4

ingredients

1 cup part-skim ricotta cheese
2 cups peaches
4 tablespoons slivered almonds
1 tablespoon maple syrup
¼ teaspoon almond extract

cooking instructions

Mix the ricotta with the maple syrup and almond extract.

Equally divide the peaches among four bowls. Top with flavored ricotta
and sprinkle the slivered almonds.

Sugar Snap Peas with Salmon

serves 4

ingredients

1 tablespoon olive oil
2 cups sugar snap peas
2 garlic cloves, minced
1 lemon
4 ounces salmon, thinly sliced
Salt and pepper to taste

cooking instructions

Remove strings along both lengths of the sugar snap peas. Heat a wok with the olive oil over medium heat. Add the garlic and sauté quickly. Add the sugar snap peas and sauté until almost tender. Add the salmon and sauté quickly. Sprinkle with lemon juice, season to taste, and serve immediately.

Tofu Cornbread

serves 8

ingredients

16 ounces soft tofu

2 eggs

3 tablespoons canola oil

¼ cup honey

1 cup instant low-fat milk powder

¼ cup whole wheat flour

½ teaspoon salt

1 ½ teaspoons baking powder

½ teaspoon baking soda

1½ cups cornmeal

2 jalapeños, finely chopped

2 ounces grated white cheddar cheese

2 tablespoons cilantro, minced

cooking instructions

Preheat the oven to 425°F.

Place the tofu, eggs, oil, honey, milk powder, flour, salt, baking powder, and baking soda in a blender. Mix until smooth. Stir in the cornmeal, jalapeños, cheese, and cilantro. Pour the mixture in an oiled pan. Bake for 25 to 30 minutes. Slice and serve immediately.

Broccoli with Pumpkin Hummus

serves 8

ingredients

2 tablespoons almond butter
2 teaspoons flaxseed oil
1 tablespoon lemon juice
1 teaspoon ground cumin
½ teaspoon ground coriander
2 cups cooked garbanzo beans
2 cups cooked pumpkin purée
1 garlic clove, pureed

1 teaspoon paprika
3 pounds broccoli
Salt to taste

cooking instructions

Combine all the ingredients, except the broccoli florets, in a food processor. Mix until very smooth and thin out with water as needed. Serve with broccoli florets.

Desserts

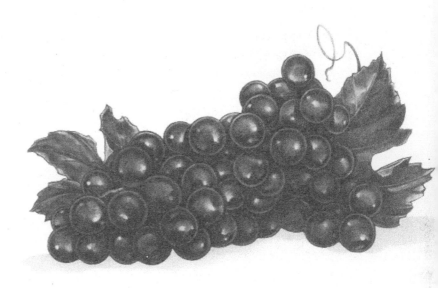

Pomegranate and Strawberry Parfait

serves 2

ingredients

1½ cups strawberries
2 ounces pure acai, no sugar added
1 teaspoon vanilla extract
1 cup low-fat Greek yogurt
2 tablespoons pomegranate seeds

cooking instructions

Mix the strawberries with vanilla extract and acai. Marinade for 30 minutes. Spoon half the fruit mixture into four parfait glasses. Top with yogurt and finish with the berries. Sprinkle with the pomegranate seeds and serve immediately.

Apple and Pear Minestrone

serves 2

ingredients

1 medium apple, brunoise
(about 5 ounces)
1 medium pear, brunoise
(about 5 ounces)
¾ cup jasmine green tea
(or your favorite)
1½ teaspoons honey

½ teaspoon pumpkin pie spices
1 small ginger root, minced
½ teaspoon lemon zest
½ teaspoon grapeseed oil

cooking instructions

Heat the oil in a deep saucepan over high heat. Add the apple and
sauté for two minutes. Add the pear, spices, ginger, lemon zest, and
sauté another minute. Add the green tea and bring to a boil. Remove
from heat and transfer to a serving bowl. Cool at room temperature.
Refrigerate for an hour or, even better, overnight to allow flavors to
emerge. Serve cold.

Baked Apples with Cranberries

serves 4
1 serving: 1 apple

ingredients

4 large apples
3 tablespoons red currant jelly
4 tablespoons cranberry juice
4 teaspoons walnuts
4 teaspoons cranberries

cooking instructions

Preheat the oven to 400°F.

Wash and core the apples, being careful not to break through the bottom of the apples. Place them in a baking pan that is just the right size to keep the apples close to eachother. Put 1 teaspoon of red currant jelly in the cavity of each apple. Pour one tablespoon of cranberry juice over the cavity of each apple. Add a little hot water in the pan (¼ inch). Cover the pan with aluminum foil and bake for 20 minutes. Remove cover and baste with the liquid in the pan. Continue baking uncovered for 4 to 5 minutes. If necessary, add a little more water to avoid burning.

Place each apple in a serving dish. Scrape particles from the pan and transfer the liquid to a saucepan. Blend the liquid with the remaining red currant jelly and bring to a boil over high heat. Pour over the apples, sprinkle with the walnuts, cranberries, and serve immediately.

Spring Fruit Salad with White Tea

serves 4

ingredients

1 small banana, sliced
3 ounces strawberries, halved
3 ounces blueberries
3 ounces raspberries
1 small apple, cubed
2 large plums, quartered
1 white tea sachet
1 tablespoon honey
1 tablespoon lemon juice

cooking instructions

Boil ¾ cup of water. Add the lemon juice, tea sachet, honey, and infuse until desired strength. Remove sachet and cool completely. Blend all the fruits in a large bowl. Add the cold tea and refrigerate for 30 minutes, mixing every 10 minutes. Serve cold.

Thin Peach and Apricot Tart

serves 8

ingredients

3 ounces almond meal

2 ounces oats

3 tablespoons grapeseed oil

Pinch of salt

1 tablespoon almond extract

2 to 3 tablespoons ice cold water

2 tablespoons apricot preserves

2 large peaches (about 8 ounces)

4 large apricots (about 8 ounces)

cooking instructions

Preheat the oven to 475°F. Place the oats in a blender and reduce to a flour consistency. Place the oat and almond flours in a bowl. Add salt, oil, almond extract, and mix until crumbly. Add one tablespoon water at a time and continue until the dough is smooth and sticks together as one ball. Lay the dough on wax paper and push down with your palm to flatten a bit. Roll out the dough to a round thin form. Then turn over the dough to a cookie sheet. Brush 1 tablespoon preserves all over the pie dough surface. Peel the peaches, apricots, and cut in half. Core, quarter, and slice. Starting at the edge of the dough and working inward toward the center, arrange the peach slices in overlapping circles. Finish with a circle of apricot slices in the center. Bake for 15 to 20 minutes until golden brown with slightly darker edges. Heat the remaining preserves in the microwave with a little water to thin. Remove the tart from the oven and brush with the peach preserves. Transfer to a cooling rack.

Fig Compote with Yogurt

serves 4

ingredients

1 cup figs
1 cup fresh orange juice
1 medium lemon peel, minced
1 medium orange peel, minced
1 fresh rosemary sprig
3 tablespoons honey
8 ounces low-fat yogurt
1 ounce walnuts, chopped

cooking instructions

Peel the figs and cut in half lengthwise. In a saucepan, combine the orange juice, peels, and rosemary. Bring to a boil over medium heat and simmer for 3 minutes. Remove the rosemary, add the figs and honey, cover, and simmer for 15 minutes. Mix, crushing the figs, and thicken for 5 minutes or to desired thickness. Beware, the mixture will thicken when cooled. Remove from heat and cool. Refrigerate for at least 2 hours before using.

Prepare 4 dessert dishes. Divide the yogurt among the dishes and top with the fig compote. Sprinkle the walnuts and serve immediately.

Red Fruit Compote

serves 4

✓ *Suggestion: Serve with low-fat yogurt, sherbet, cream of millet, apple slices, etc.*

ingredients

8 ounces blackberries
8 ounces raspberries
8 ounces blueberries
8 ounces strawberries
3 tablespoons honey
1 large organic lemon peel

1 large organic orange peel
1 cup pomegranate juice
(no sugar added)
Cornstarch mixed with a little water

cooking instructions

Wash the berries and carefully pat dry. Place the pomegranate juice in a saucepan and bring to boil over high heat. Reduce by half. If necessary, thicken with a little water-cornstarch mixture. Add the honey, berries, and cook for a minute or two. Do not overcook, or you will end up with a sauce rather than a compote. Remove from heat and transfer the compote to a bowl. Place the bowl in an ice-cold water bath to stop the cooking process. Refrigerate for two hours before serving.

Peach with Apricot Coulis

serves 8

ingredients

4 peaches
12 apricots
1 tablespoon honey
1 teaspoon lemon juice
1 rosemary branch
4 teaspoons almonds

cooking instructions

Cut apricots in half and remove pits. Place the apricots in a pan. Add ½ cup water, honey, rosemary, lemon juice, and bring to a boil. Reduce heat, cover, and simmer for ten minutes. Purée in a blender and transfer to a serving bowl. Let cool and refrigerate. Peel and cut the peaches in half. Place the peach halves on a serving platter, drizzle with some apricot sauce and the almonds. Serve with the remaining apricot sauce on the side.

Fruit Salad with Mint

serves 4

✓ *As an alternative, you can try substituting white or green tea leaves for the mint leaves in this recipe.*

ingredients

1 tablespoon lemon juice
1 mint tea sachet
1 tablespoon honey
1 small banana, sliced
3 ounces strawberries, halved
3 ounces blueberries

3 ounces raspberries
1 small apple, cubed
2 large plums, pitted and quartered
2 tablespoons chopped fresh mint leaves
¼ cup pomegranate seeds

cooking instructions

Boil ¾ cup water. Add the lemon juice, tea sachet, and honey, and infuse to desired strength. Remove sachet and cool completely.

Mix all the fruits in a large bowl. Add the cold tea and refrigerate for 30 minutes, mixing every 10 minutes. Mix in the fresh mint and pomegranate, then serve immediately.

Marie's Oatmeal Cookies

20 cookies

ingredients

7 ounces almond meal
¾ cup brown sugar
1½ teaspoons baking powder
¾ teaspoon baking soda
¼ teaspoon salt

1 extra large egg
2 ounces apricot preserves
1 cup Old Fashioned
Quaker® Oats
2 ounces unsalted butter

cooking instructions

Preheat the oven to 350°F. Prepare a couple of cookie sheets covered with a silpat mat or parchment paper. Mix the almond meal, brown sugar, baking powder, baking soda, and salt. Blend in the egg and the preserves. Melt the butter and let cool for a minute. Add the oats to the almond mixture and mix well. Add the melted butter. Scoop out the dough with a #30 scoop (about 1 ounce cookie) onto the cookie sheet, placing the mounds 3 inches apart to allow for spreading. Refrigerate for 30 minutes. Flatten the dough slightly with your palm and bake for 12 minutes or until golden brown. Let cool in the pan before transferring to a cooling rack.

This type of cookie will be moist. Don't store for more than 2 days at room temperature. It absorbs moisture quickly and can become very soggy. The best way to store them would be to freeze immediately after they cool down. Defrost at room temperature as needed or quickly defrost in the microwave for 5 to 7 seconds.

You may add ½ cup of raisins, dried fruits, coconut, chocolate chips, chopped dates, nuts, or a combination of various ingredients. Remember, any of these ingredients will add calories to the original recipe.

You may also add 1 teaspoon cinnamon and/or ½ teaspoon allspice.

Marie's Chocolate Oatmeal Cookies: Reduce almond meal to 6 ounces and add ⅓ cup pure cocoa powder. Follow the same direction as recipe above. Add the cocoa powder with the oats.

Pears with Roquefort Cheese

✓ *If Roquefort is not available, substitute with Gorgonzola.*

serves 4

ingredients

4 pears, sliced
4 ounces Roquefort cheese, crumbled
4 tablespoons chopped walnuts

cooking instructions

Divide the pears among four plates. Sprinkle with the cheese, walnuts, and serve immediately.

Stuffed Peaches

serves 4

ingredients

4 peaches, washed and patted dry
4 to 5 amaretti cookies
1 teaspoon minced orange peel
1 tablespoon honey
1 large egg white
2 tablespoons blanched almonds, chopped

2 teaspoons butter, in 8 pats
½ cup white Muscat
¼ cup water

cooking instructions

Preheat the oven to 375°F.

Cut the peaches in half and remove the pits. Scoop out a little bit of the flesh from the center. Finely chop the scooped flesh and place in a bowl. Crush the cookies and add to the bowl. Mix in the orange peel, honey, egg white, and almonds. Spoon the mixture equally into the peach halves. Top with a small pat of butter. Place the stuffed peaches in a baking pan, add the wine and water, and bake for about 25 to 30 minutes. Serve immediately.

Baked Apples with Pomegranate Preserves

> ✓ *Option: Substitute pomegranate preserves with currant or raspberry preserves.*

serves 4, 1 serving: 1 apple

ingredients

4 teaspoons walnuts
4 large apples
9 teaspoons pomegranate preserves
4 tablespoons pomegranate juice
4 tablespoons pomegranate seeds

cooking instructions

Preheat the broiler. Cover the bottom of a baking sheet with parchment paper. Add the walnuts and broil until slightly browned. Remove from the sheet, cool, and chop.

Preheat the oven to 400°F.

Wash and core the apples, being careful not to break through the bottom of the apples. Place them in a baking pan that is just the right size to keep the apples close to each other. Put 1 teaspoon of pomegranate preserves in the cavity of each apple. Pour 1 tablespoon of pomegranate juice into the cavity of each apple. Add a little hot water to the pan (about ¼ inch high). Cover the pan with aluminum foil and bake for 20 minutes. Remove foil and baste with the pan liquids. Continue baking uncovered for 4 to 5 minutes. If necessary, add a little more water to avoid burning.

Place each apple in a serving dish. Scrape particles from the pan and transfer the liquid to a saucepan. Blend the liquid with the remaining pomegranate preserves and bring to boil over high heat. Pour over the apples, sprinkle the walnuts, pomegranate seeds, and serve immediately.

Fresh Figs
with Cinnamon Butter

serves 4

✔ *Serve the figs with your favorite sherbert, plain yogurt, or even Pecorino shavings.*

ingredients

2 tablespoons unsalted butter
2 tablespoons grapeseed oil
3 tablespoons honey
½ teaspoon ground cinnamon
8 fresh figs, cut in half

cooking instructions

Melt the butter without disturbing it over low heat. Once melted, skim off the white particles floating on the surface. Add the oil, honey, and cinnamon. Mix until dissolved. Add the figs halves and brown on both sides. Serve the figs immediately.

Carrot Cake

serves 12

ingredients

One 21-ounce package of Pamela's™ Classic Vanilla Cake Mix
1 teaspoon baking soda
2 teaspoons cinnamon
¾ teaspoon cloves
½ teaspoon ginger
½ teaspoon nutmeg
1 teaspoon vanilla
3 large eggs

¼ cup grapeseed oil
½ cup water
1 cup shredded carrots
½ cup chopped walnuts
½ cup plump raisins
1 cup crushed pineapple, juice removed
½ cup sweetened shredded coconut
Powdered sugar

cooking instructions

Preheat the oven to 350°F. Lightly grease a 9-x-13-inch pan.

In a bowl, mix the cake mix and baking soda. Add the spices, vanilla, eggs, oil, and water, and mix until incorporated. Fold in the carrots, walnuts, raisins, pineapple, and coconut. Transfer to the pan and bake for 30 to 35 minutes or until a toothpick inserted in the center comes out clean. Let cool in the pan. Transfer to a serving platter and sprinkle powdered sugar.

Pumpkin Harvest Bread with Ice Cream

serves 16

ingredients

1½ cups flour
½ cup cornmeal
1½ teaspoons baking powder
1 teaspoon baking soda
¼ teaspoon salt
2 teaspoons ground cinnamon
½ teaspoon ground nutmeg
1 cup solid pack cooked pumpkin
(fresh or from organic can)

2 eggs
1 cup packed brown sugar
¼ cup vegetable oil
¼ cup apricot preserves
½ cup raisins
½ cup walnuts
4 cups low-fat vanilla ice cream

cooking instructions

Preheat the oven to 350°F.

Combine the flour, cornmeal, baking powder, baking soda, salt, cinnamon, and nutmeg in a bowl. Beat the pumpkin, eggs, brown sugar, oil and preserves in a large mixing bowl. Incorporate the flour mixture and blend until well mixed. Stir in the raisins, walnuts, and transfer to a greased and floured loaf pan. Bake for 50 to 55 minutes or until wooden pick inserted into the center comes out clean. Cool in pan for 5 to 10 minutes. Transfer the loaf to a wire rack and cool completely before slicing. Serve each slice with ¼ cup low-fat vanilla ice cream.

References

Online Resources:

The Mayo Clinic
www.mayoclinic.com

National Cancer Institute
www.cancer.gov/cancertopics/types/prostate4

National Kidney and Urological Diseases Clearinghouse (NKUDIC)
www.kidney.niddk.nih.gov

World Foundation of Urology NGO
www.prostatecancerprevention.net

My Recipes

My Recipes

_____

_____

_____

_____

_____

_____

_____

_____

_____

_____

_____

_____

_____

_____

_____

_____

_____

_____

_____

My Recipes

My Recipes

My Recipes

My Recipes